This journal belongs to: _____

If found, please contact: _____

SWEET-ASS JOURNAL
TO OPTIMIZE YOUR
DIABETIC LIFESTYLE

in 100 Days

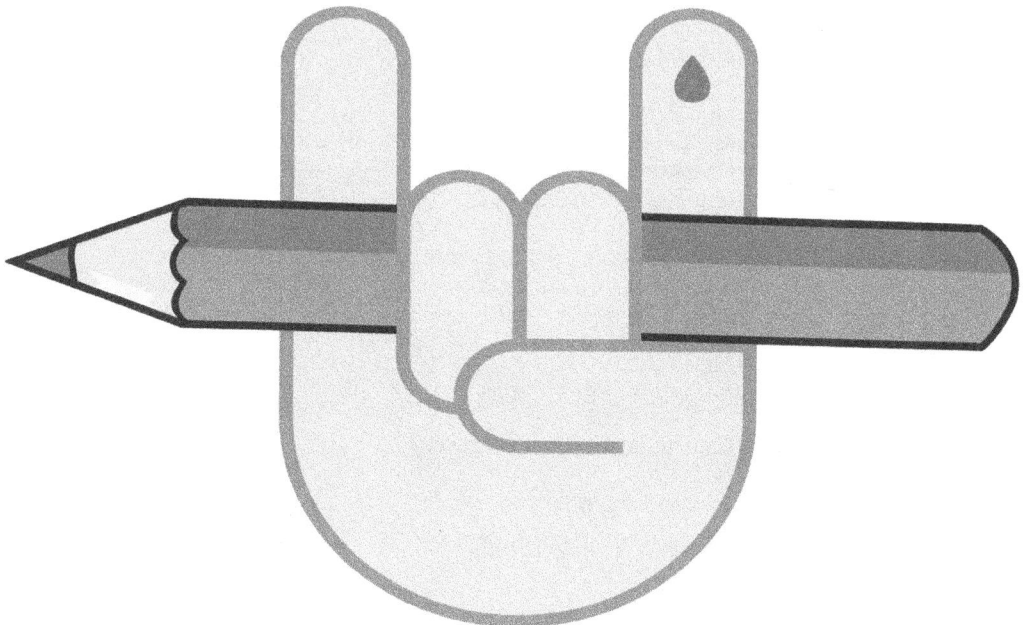

Disclaimer

The information provided within this publication is for general informational purposes only. While we try to keep the information up-to-date and correct, there are no representations or warranties, express or implied, about the completeness, accuracy, reliability, suitability or availability with respect to the information, products, services, or related graphics contained in this publication for any purpose. Any use of this information is at your own risk.

The methods described within this guide and journal are the author's personal thoughts, recommendations, and experiences. They are not intended to be a definitive set of instructions for this project. You may discover there are other methods and materials to accomplish the same end result. You may also discover that the author's methods do not generate the same results for you. Either way, you're still a champion.

The authors do not assume and hereby disclaim any liability to any party for any loss, damage, or disruption caused by errors or omissions, whether such errors or omissions result from accident, negligence, or any other cause. If you wish to apply ideas contained in this publication, you are taking full responsibility for your actions.

All information, content, and material in this journal and all content affiliated is for informational purposes only and is not intended to serve as a substitute for the consultation, diagnosis, and/or medical treatment by a qualified physician or healthcare provider.

Copyright

ISBN: 978-1-7342329-1-2
Designed by Heath Armstrong and Caitlin Grenier
Edited by Lily Ann Fouts

© Copyright 2020 Fist Pumps LLC and CRMG LLC, Heath Armstrong and Caitlin Grenier
All Rights Reserved (for pizza parties too)
Published by Heath Armstrong and Caitlin Grenier

No part of this publication may be reproduced or transmitted in any form or by any means, electronic or mechanical, including photocopying, recording or by any information storage and retrieval system, without written permission from the publisher and author.

For inquiries about permissions for reproducing parts of this guide and journal, please e-mail:

partylikeadiabetic@gmail.com or **heath@fistpumps.com**

For more information, visit the authors' websites at:

www.partylikeadiabetic.co or **www.heatharmstrong.com**

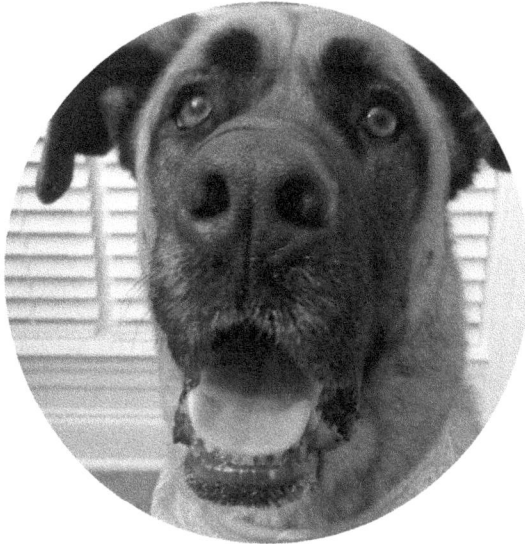

Dedication

To Loki Anne Armstrong, for sharing your angelic singing voice at all times, no matter what forces tried to suppress my happiness. You are my eternal reminder to smile, without reason or expectation. Without your lucky Lokes ears, these sustainable happiness practices would not be a part of my life. Aho, silly Lokes.

-Love, Heath

To all the warriors who fight the silent battle against diabetes and never give up. To everyone that gives it their all, no matter how difficult. To anyone who has to say "I have diabetes." Much love, my friends.

-Caitlin

SWEET-ASS CONTENTS

Part 1: Setting the Stage 15
Becoming Something More 17
A Quick Note on Resistance Gremlins 18
Kickstarting the Habit and Tracking Momentum 19
Sweet-Ass 100-Day Vision 19
The Mosaic Journal Layout 21

Part 2: Overview of Journal Sections 23
AM and PM 25
Morning Quotes for Fist Pumping 25
Blood Glucose Tracker 25
Breath of Life 26
Sweet-Ass Affirmations 28
Morning Sections Guide 33
Most-Valuable Daily Actions 35
Big Cheese 37
Sweet-Ass Reward 39
Wildcard Box 39
Evening Sections Guide 41
Winning 43
Party Checklist 45
Planning Ahead: Tomorrow's Most Valuable Daily Actions 46
Reflection and Thoughts 47

Part 3: The Journal 49
Time to Party and Never Give Up 51
Example of Completed Journal 53
Optimize Your Diabetic Lifestyle in 100 Days 57
Exercise and Movement — Show that Beautiful Body Some Love 72
Sweet-Ass Affirmation Cards 80
Creating Your Sacred Space 84
Meal Planning and Nutrition Optimization 92
7-Day Giving Challenge 106
Sweet-Ass 100-Day Visions: Quarterly Review 1 118
Abundance Lists 126
Brainstorming Ideas 142
Experience Challenges 162
Sweet-Ass 100-Day Visions: Quarterly Review 2 180
10-Day Minimalist Challenge — Removing Physical and Digital Distractions 186
Sweet-Ass 100-Day Visions: Quarterly Review 3 238
Sweet-Ass Finish Line 295
Special Invitation to Connect 297

BONUS MATERIAL DOWNLOADS

You can download all bonus material mentioned throughout this journal by visiting:

www.sweetassjournal.com/pladbonus

Introduction: The Sweet-Ass Journal Origin

Heath Armstrong

In the Winter of 2016, I walked downstairs to a cold, eerie basement that I had come to know as my sacred creative space in a small house I was renting in Walla Walla, Washington. As I edged closer to the bottom step, something seemed off with the smell of the air. The stack of journaling systems I was using to hold my life together was also in complete disarray, as if it had come to life and was loudly screaming "Dude, why did you let this happen to me?!"

It took me a couple of seconds to figure out what had happened, but once I did, I immediately fell face forward into the dark pit of terror and madness. How could this have happened? NOOO! WHY!!!!???

I'll get back to that in a minute.

Just five years earlier, after starting my night with a few beers at some random Octoberfest celebration in Lexington, Kentucky, I woke up face-down-pants-down on my garage floor at around 9:00 a.m. Just inches from the wooden steps leading into the house, my nose had been leaking blood onto the concrete floor, and my hand still grasped an empty bottle of Jim Beam that I must have acquired somewhere along the way.

I was too weak to approach and turn off my car, still running, parked in the middle of the front yard as though abandoned in a high-speed chase after a Cops episode.

A few years later, in February 2014, I woke up yet again from another night of blackout numbness. Although I hated myself for the situations, I couldn't seem to break the habit. I pulled myself down to the oversized jacuzzi tub in my excessive four-bedroom house with five televisions, a full bar and too many fish tanks to count, and I just hit the floor in shambles. I cried. I pulled my hair out. I held my breath underwater and considered making the pain go away forever. The army of fear and resistance had me at check-mate, and I knew I had to make changes if I wanted to get out alive.

But, how?

Under the guidance of a few special people that trickled into my life (Amber Vilhauer, Hal Elrod, Paul Kemp), I decided to start interviewing happy and successful people around the world who were living passionately, no matter what harsh situations the world presented them with. My goal was to highlight any commonalities in their habits, approach, and lifestyle and see what would happen if I applied them to my life.

It wasn't long before the number of interviews capped the 100 mark, and the habits and strategies I learned and started applying to my life helped me make a mass transformation that still doesn't seem real.

In just two and a half years, I:

- Sold my house and everything I owned to eliminate distractions and discover meaning.
- Paid off over $20,000 in personal debt.
- Retired my 'traditional career' in exchange for my own passionate, purposeful projects.
- Automated a high-revenue e-commerce business and became my own boss.
- Moved to the Pacific Northwest as I had always dreamed of doing.
- Started traveling the world, testing my comfort zone in the best ways possible.

All these changes were catapulted off the back of one very simple change: **the introduction of personal daily habits to improve mindset, health, and happiness.**

After discovering the personal daily habits that fueled all the incredible people I interviewed, I was neurotically tracking them all in separate journals like a mad scientist on speed. I had thoughts about making the system more simple, and possibly sharing the ideas with others, but I was too scared and full of resistance to step into that light.

As I got to the bottom of the steps in that cold, eerie basement, the horrid smell and disorganized terror revealed itself! My handsome black lab, Arlonious Bologna Maximus, had lifted his leg and let down a stream of his own glory to soak all my journals. Not only that, he had jaw-chomped a few into unrecognizable pieces. The rage consumed me! All my sensitive, important information was soiled!

Just a few hours later, I remembered back to a year or so earlier when I had a call with my coach at the time, Jacqueline du Plessis. She said, "Dude, why don't you just put all of those systems into one simple journal that other people can use too? You want to be a writer, right? You have to start."

She was right. I've always wanted to be a writer, and I've also always wanted to help others overcome any resistance, fears, or situations that are keeping them from ultimate happiness as well. I don't want anyone to feel like I used to feel, ever. I did just as she suggested.

In early 2017, I released *The Sweet Ass Journal to Develop Your Happiness Muscle in 100 Days*. I had no idea what kind of impact it would have on my life, let alone the thousands of wonderful souls that would end up using it. Since its release, I've had hundreds of beautiful people reach out about the effect the journal is having on their mindset, health, and overall happiness. Most of the transitions and stories people have shared with me have brought genuine tears, outrageous laughs, and pure gratitude to my creative path.

Meeting Caitlin

One of the beautiful and brilliant people I met along the way was Caitlin Grenier, the co-author of this journal. Caitlin is a diabetic, and she embraces every bit of the journey. She glows with happiness and health. We met through a lunch meeting with my sister in Nashville, Tennessee in 2018, and she expressed to me her life mission to help diabetics optimize their lifestyles, mindsets, and overall health. As I shared the journal with her, we immediately noticed a huge chunk of practices that could be beneficial to diabetics, as most of them positively impact stress and happiness levels, which can in return have an astonishing effect on keeping blood glucose levels in range and steady.

At this point, I had almost two years of great feedback from *The Sweet Ass Journal to Develop Your Happiness Muscle in 100 Days*, as well as further research into the science of WHY these practices work. I had already started working on a revised version of the original journal, and I was instantly intrigued by Caitlin's mission. When she asked, half joking, if we could make a version of the journal specifically for diabetics, excitement flooded my creative brain.

So, here we are! Party!

Caitlin and I have spent countless hours to make this system simple, enjoyable, and exciting for you. In a moment, she is going to share her heart with you, and then we will dive into the journal sections and how they work.

Big love!

-Heath

Introduction: Party Like A Diabetic

Caitlin Grenier

"Webbie, you don't understand. I NEED to find a fruit smoothie. I don't care where we have to drive to find one and how much I have to pay." This desperate person was me talking with my fellow graduate student and research partner in August 2013 while we were in the field conducting our thesis research on halibut parasitology and growth (totally cool when you live in Alaska). At the time, I was having horrible cravings for sweets, carbs, and fruit. You would think that a fruit smoothie would not be difficult to find, but when you are in the fishing town of Homer, Alaska, that is not the case. Webbie was a trooper, though, and walked all over with me until we found something that resembled a fruit smoothie. I literally cannot describe how excited I was about this. As soon as the barista handed over the 16-ounce strawberry banana cup of frozen heaven I received a phone call from my doctor.

Why would I be getting a personal call from my doctor? Well, a week before this call I was at my parents' house, and while walking down the stairs, I randomly got blurry vision and almost stumbled the whole way down. I walked into the kitchen and finally admitted to my mom that I needed to go to the doctor. There was something very wrong with me. I had been having symptoms for months, but as a graduate student working two jobs, I thought it was just stress. I had rapidly lost about 35 pounds without trying, was drinking gallons of water a day without being satiated, peeing an insane amount throughout the day and night, experiencing muscle cramps, sleeping as much as I possibly could but still feeling exhausted, having blurry vision, slurring my speech, and feeling cravings like never before. Looking back, I just have to shake my head about how obvious it was.

Back to the smoothie in Homer, Alaska, though. I had just taken my first glorious, satisfying sip when my doctor said, "We got your blood work back and it looks like you are diabetic. You need to stay away from carbs like bread, sugar, and fruit." My face went completely blank, I put the smoothie down and reluctantly slid it across the table to Webbie who at that point was incredibly confused, and rightly so. "Cait, we just spent an hour and a half looking for that and you are giving it to me?" I was in shock. I was in denial. I was not ready to hear that.

I kept thinking this had to be temporary and it would go away with more exercise, better nutrition, supplements, vitamins, anything. I was so convinced and determined to FIX this. My primary care physician (PCP) referred me to an endocrinologist in town, and when I sat down in his office a week later I got a dose of reality. He started talking about the test results and told me that I had late-onset type 1 diabetes and that I would have to start taking insulin. Due to my shock and confusion I asked him, "Ok, how long will I have to be on insulin for?" I kid you not, he laughed at me and said, "Forever." At that point, I broke down. I was not ready to hear that or comprehend what life would be like now. Thank God my mom was with me to help me through this process. I still remember that doctor visit vividly, and likely will never forget it.

You may be able to guess what came next. Yes — depression, more weight loss, and most of all, anger and fear. I had amazing support from friends and family, and while I knew they cared, they didn't directly understand what I was going through. How could they?

So I found myself facing two choices: let diabetes control me, or find a way to control it. I started reaching out to other diabetics, went to seminars, heard others' stories, and then gained the courage to share my own. This led to a new career path addressing diabetes prevention for the YMCA and becoming a National Board Certified Health and Wellness Coach specializing in healthcare professionals and diabetics through Vanderbilt. But I still had a thirst to do more. Being an extrovert, foodie, dancer, lover of wine, and social butterfly, I was tired of guessing carbs and how much medication I had to take to enjoy all the parts of life I wanted to indulge in. I was tired of feeling misunderstood and alone. I was tired of the worry and added stress of my new normal. What could I do to make this new normal easier? Over a beer with my sister, we spouted ideas off each other until the phrase "Party Like A Diabetic" rolled off our tongues. This is it. This is an avenue for me to make a difference, not just for myself, but for everyone who has ever had to say out loud: "I have diabetes."

Whether you have type 1, type 2, LADA, MODY or prediabetes, we are positive that the information and processes in this journal, along with the amazing online Party Like A Diabetic community, will help you live your best life!

<3 -Caitlin

Taking Charge

To reach optimal health and happiness, first acknowledge you need to make changes. Then be relentless in manifesting these changes. Our goal with this Sweet-Ass Journal is to help you stay focused on the magic of life in the moment, so you can use all moments to efficiently create and sustain a low-stress life of optimal health, happiness, and purpose forever.

If you take only one step toward completing a section of this journal daily, then EVERY day you are moving in the direction of your vision, personal development, and ultimate happiness and freedom.

Even though we designed this journal to optimize your diabetic lifestyle and increase your happiness, we also aim for it to be a shortcut to kickstart and track the magical journey you are about to embark upon for the rest of your life. The journal is not meant to be overwhelming, so don't feel anxious or stressed if you miss a few sections or days. We both fall off track often, but it's always there to pick back up when we need it the most.

In the following sections of this journal, you will learn powerful daily habits that will fuel your optimal lifestyle, such as deep breathing, affirming visions, priority focusing, practicing gratitude, tracking health, giving gifts, minimizing distractions, brainstorming ideas, celebrating wins, planning ahead, and reflecting.

We promise you'll laugh, too... :)

PART 1:

SETTING THE STAGE

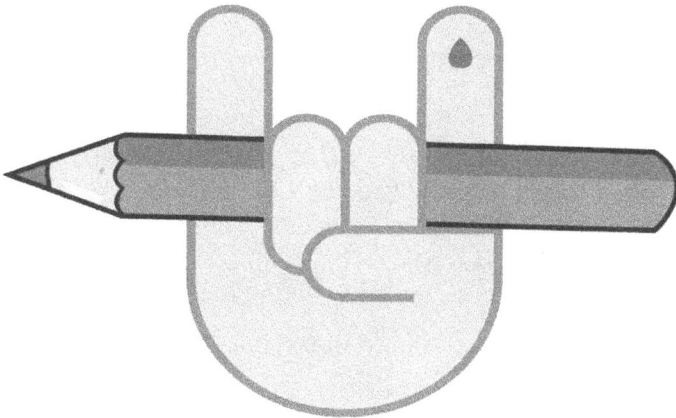

Becoming Something More

As with any journey in life, you should aim for something more. Every moment of every day, we want to support you in progressing toward a happier, healthier, and more valuable self. Take action during your days to ensure you are a better person when your head hits the pillow than you were upon rising that morning.

Use this journal persistently, and you may notice a magical transformation similar to the ones we have experienced, as well as thousands of other amazing people who have used these journaling systems. We are not suggesting that by filling out a page of this journal every once in awhile you will become superhuman with the answers to all of life. However, if you use this journal with the fire and grit to become one with the elevation that awaits within you, there is a good chance you'll learn how to:

- Set a vision for your 100-day transformation. Stop the guesswork and know where you want to be and how you want to feel at the end of your 100 days!
- Kickstart your days with deep breathing, followed by positive affirmations to bring your visions to reality.
- Identify and achieve your most valuable daily actions to consistently move toward your goals, dreams, and optimal health. No more wasted time on meaningless goober tasks.
- Digest a breakfast of smiles and gratitude. Wrap your brain around positive vibes to shape the rest of your day.
- Manage and track your diet, exercise routines, and water intake.
- Manage and track your blood sugars in order to see trends throughout your day and over time.
- Reward yourself for everything you accomplish. You deserve it!
- Become a master of brainstorming ideas, some of which will change your life!

- Eliminate emotional and physical distractions and surround yourself with value and support. Less is more.
- Bring back and sustain that warm, fuzzy feeling you had as a child. Remember that sweet-ass feeling?
- Celebrate your progress to optimize motivation and excitement.
- Plan your magical day the night before to clear your mind while you sleep.
- Reflect upon your progress, thoughts, and experiences of your journey.
- Beef up your happiness muscle and optimize your diabetic lifestyle!

These practices and habits will contribute to lower stress, a calmer mind, and elevated happiness. It's almost time to start your transformation and set your vision, but first, a few more insights to help you get the party started!

A Quick Note on Resistance Gremlins

You may see this phrase throughout the journal and in most of Heath's work, so it deserves a brief explanation. We experience the monster of resistance in our lifelong battle to create our freedom and happiness empires. Some of the more common forms of resistance are fear, stress, anxiety, and procrastination. Brilliant authors and philosophers have dissected resistance in their work since the beginning of literacy (Steven Pressfield's *The War of Art* being a recent example), and there is good reason for this. Resistance is the enemy of creation. If we can identify it and suppress it, we can create magic.

When we resist, we conform to the death of creation—the death of ourselves. When we create, we destroy resistance. Obviously, to manifest an optimal life of pure happiness and elevated health, we must create it. Therefore, we must destroy resistance.

Everyone experiences resistance, but not everyone can identify the beast. It can creep into life in disguise as comfort, assurance, and even family and friends. So, it's immensely important to be able to identify resistance, and then take all actions necessary to contain, suppress, and beat it down!

If we attach "gremlin" to the back of resistance, it makes it easier for us to understand that resistance is a real crippling energy that lives to dismantle our creations and hinder our progress. Then, we can personify anything that stands in our way by attaching a gremlin face and body to it. In our world, there are email gremlins, insulin gremlins, carb gremlins, insurance gremlins, testing gremlins, Doctor appointment gremlins, Facebook gremlins, alcohol gremlins, weather gremlins, sleep gremlins, exercise gremlins, focus gremlins, and even travel gremlins! These nasty little goons can show up anywhere, anytime, in any form, and it's not only humorous to envision them with gremlin heads, but it directly helps to keep the focus on identifying and destroying anything that stands in the way of our persistence and personal creative development.

Resistance gremlins are your enemy. Keep your weapons sharp and make those evil little creatures afraid of you! You are a dia-badass! You have important work to do!

Kickstarting the Habit and Tracking Momentum

Your new journal is laid out in 100 days and nights to make it incredibly easy to track your progress. Because there are 100 days of journaling, each page represents 1% of 100%. Therefore, if you complete your journal on day one, you are 1% to completing your 100 days of optimizing your diabetic lifestyle! If you wrap up entry 98, you'll be 98% finished with pumping that diabetic lifestyle into fully optimal shape! And we can attest, each day that you complete will be a step toward ultimate happiness and freedom. You can always see what percent you have completed by checking the bottom right-hand corner of the journal.

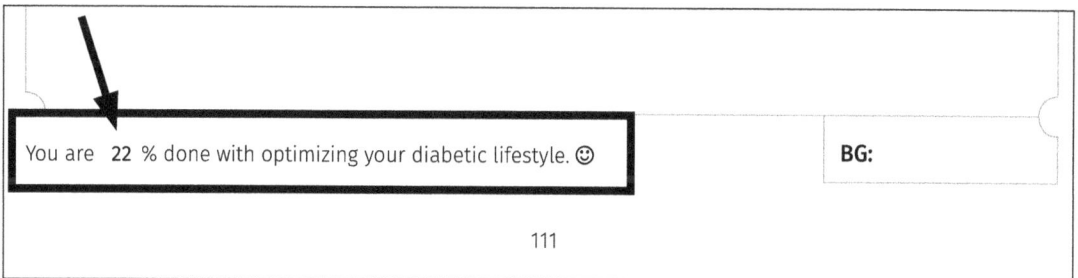

You are 22 % done with optimizing your diabetic lifestyle. ☺	BG:

111

Sweet-Ass 100-Day Vision

Set Your 100-Day Goals for Achieving Optimal Happiness and Health

Before you start this journey, it's important to visualize who you wish to become in this process. By creating a vision, you are setting a focus for where you are heading in life. If you follow the direction of your vision, you create a path directly to it. If you fail to create your own vision, others will make your vision for you by placing ads, commercials, billboards, politics, traditions, and rules all around you. Do yourself a monstrous favor and define your future without these outside influences!

Since you have this journal in your hand, you are already taking action to build the future you. On the next page, write down three visions (AKA goals or dreams) that you wish to bloom between now and the 100 awesome days of this ride. These can be health goals, business goals, lifestyle goals, or perhaps one of each—as long as they are in alignment with the most optimal version of yourself. Aim high! Coming up short on a big scary goal is better than accomplishing one with minimal effort. Prepare to achieve one (or all) of your visions before the 100-day journaling is complete. Celebrate! Treat yourself to a super tasty night out! Then, keep hustling toward your other visions and set a new one in place of the one you have brought to reality. You will have a chance to review and modify your visions, if needed, throughout the 100-day journey.

It's important to write your visions as if they are happening or have already happened. When you repeat them out loud, you want to speak about them like they are part of your current life. This helps affirm to your subconscious mind that these manifestations are taking place. The more you affirm your vision to your mind, the more you'll subconsciously make decisions (without even thinking about them) to move toward your visions and your dreams.

Here are some examples to get your mind jogging:

- I have reduced my A1c by 0.6% and sustained the new level.
- I have no diabetic complications.
- I sponsor at least one full scholarship a year for Diabetes Training Camp.
- I have a thriving exercise routine and have lost 15 pounds.
- I saved enough money to come to Africa and help a non-profit.
- I have an enjoyable exercise routine and have lost 15 lbs, reducing my body fat by 8%.
- I have finished the outline and rough draft of my first novel.
- I have "time in range" above 75%.
- The side business I created is making me an extra $300/month.
- I completed my first 5k run.
- I am spearheading research on stress management for diabetics to create much-needed resources (like this journal).
- I have supportive calls with a family member or friend every day on the phone.
- My sales accounts have increased at work by 20%.
- I have grown the Party Like A Diabetic online community to over 5,000 dia-badasses.
- I speak fluent Spanish.
- I sold my house, and I currently live in the Pacific Northwest.
- Party Like A Diabetic is now in every major city of the United States.

- I have paid off my credit card debt in full. Freedom!
- I have helped change the negative stigma surrounding diabetes.

Your turn!

My sweet-ass visions are:

- ....
- ....
- ....

Again, by framing these in the present tense, you store a vision in your mind of what you aim to become. In the upcoming pages, you'll learn how to set and reflect on the most valuable actions to complete each day toward realizing your visions.

Eventually, you will reach a day when your visions are a reality. We aren't promising that every vision you set will come true. If you write "I am brewing beer on the moon," it's likely this vision won't come true. But if you set reasonable goals that you believe in and care about, and you work toward them every day through your most valuable actions, you will eventually bring them to reality.

You can download and print a reminder of your visions to post on your wall and keep you on track (along with all other bonus material) at:

www.sweetassjournal.com/pladbonus.

The Mosaic Journal Layout

Everyone has a different style for journaling. Some people go looney tunes and black out the entire page with notes and ink, and others have a simple approach. Sometimes our writing is huge and lowercase as if we had never made it out of first grade, and other times our writing is neat, small, and in all caps. Sometimes it's more fun to just draw our ideas rather than write them. It all depends on our energy level and creative mood at the moment.

Because we are all unique in our approach and there is no wrong way to journal, we (with the help of the creative eye of Jacqueline du Plessis) decided on a different layout for the pages. Instead of using a traditional and fixed horizontal line layout, which can actually make us feel overwhelmed if we don't fill all the lines, we laid out this journal in free space mosaic boxes. These boxes become best friends for those who love to write big, small, messy, clean, extensive and simple. They even act as a perfect canvas for all you creative doodlers out there! It does not matter if you write one-word answers, essays, or draw a picture of your booty! Don't be overwhelmed. Just move forward.

PART 2:

OVERVIEW OF JOURNAL SECTIONS

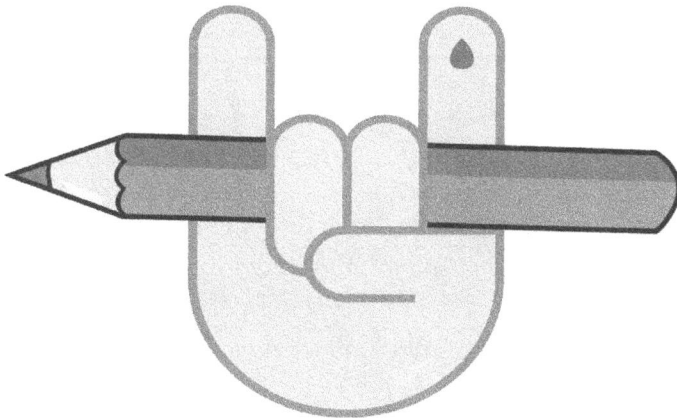

AM and PM

This journal is divided into two sections: morning and evening. The morning section sets the right mood and energy for the day, while the evening section fosters reflection on your progress and optimizes your mindset before rest. There are no direct rules as to when you must fill out the journal. Sometimes, you may find yourself filling out the night section the following morning. The idea is to visit this journal twice a day, with time in between to awaken and optimize your happiness and lifestyle.

For guaranteed progress, honor persistence.

First we will cover the sections that appear in both the morning and evening, and then we will break down the individual boxes that appear in either the AM or PM sections.

Morning Quotes for Fist Pumping

At the top of every journal entry, there is a new quote or mantra for inspiration. Read these quotes out loud while you pump your fists in the air both in the morning and in the evening! Each one of them has a personal connection to helping us in our journeys, and we trust they will inspire and help you, too!

Blood Glucose Tracker

There are two spaces in the journal each day for logging your blood glucose levels. Because these habits and practices will ultimately lower your stress and increase your happiness, it's likely your blood glucose levels will become lower and more steady as you implement these practices. In the top right corner of the morning section, just below the quote, you'll notice a box for entering your BG. It's best to record that level before you start the AM part of your journal.

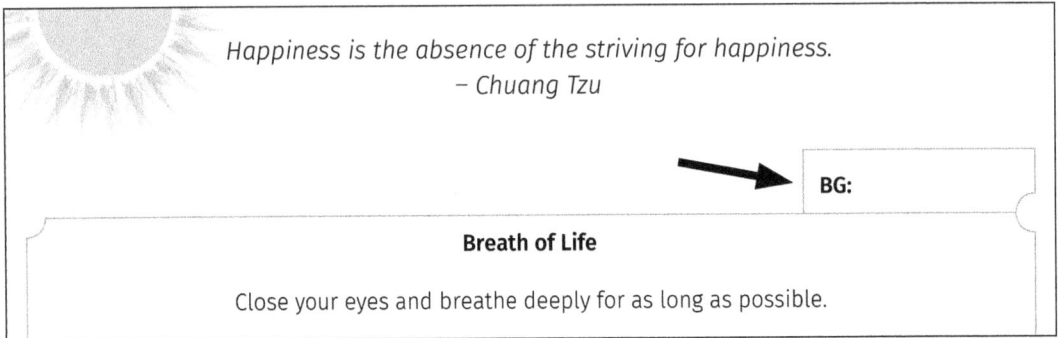

> *Happiness is the absence of the striving for happiness.*
> *– Chuang Tzu*

BG:

Breath of Life

Close your eyes and breathe deeply for as long as possible.

When you return to your journal in the evening and finish your practices and reflection for the day, you'll notice a space to record your BG in the bottom right corner. The last thing you do should be to record your level in the evening. This will give you an overview of your BG throughout the day and also help you go to bed at a safe level.

Breath of Life

Near the beginning of both the AM and PM sections, you will notice a **Breath of Life** box. This space is of high importance because your breath, in conjunction with your heartbeat, is the rhythm of your life.

By introducing occasional periods of deep breathing to your day, you can keep your brilliant mind at its highest power, allowing you to not only focus on the parts of life that matter most, but also destroy any stress gremlins that attempt to cloud the way.

Deep breathing is commonly referred to as "meditation," but the term "meditation" may show up with a heavy feeling of resistance to you. It's easy to think of meditation like the hilarious scene from *Ace Ventura: When Nature Calls*, when Jim Carrey is exaggeratedly chanting "Alrighty Then" like Brahman, the Hindu Deity, and is fully possessing his body with a surge of OM vibrations.

Vibrations, chakras, yoni eggs, astral projections, and sound baths are all super cool, but these deep and trendy practices do not have to make breathing intimidating for you.

The Breath of Life space is simply an area for you to establish a habit of periodically disconnecting from the fast-paced modern world to close your eyes and reconnect with your breath—the rhythm of life. The time range is completely open for your preference, but we encourage you to build toward longer and deeper sessions as your 100-day journey grows. Start with a couple of minutes and work your way up! Who knows, maybe soon you'll be chanting "Alrighty Then" in a random hut in the Himalayas.

If you are thinking, "Oh no, I hate meditation. I've tried it. My mind just races and it gives me anxiety, and I can't stop thinking about all the stuff I need to do," then good. You are the type of person that will benefit the most from breathing deeply (it leads to extreme relaxation, you big silly goose).

Here are a few benefits you can achieve from deep breathing:

- Lower stress and anxiety
- Calmer mind with more clarity
- Increased oxygen levels to your brain and nervous system
- Lower blood pressure
- Increased energy (yep)
- Increased mood
- Better sleep
- Pain relief
- Stronger immune system
- Balanced emotions

A few tips and ways to get started are:

- Find or create a quiet space where you feel comfortable and removed from distractions (we will introduce a process for creating your sacred space later in this journal).
- Sit or lay down comfortably.
- Put on some soft mindful or classical music in the background, or simply tune into the noise of your surroundings and nature.
- Check out the Insight Meditation Timer app for Apple or Android for free guided meditations, music, meditation timer, tracking your practice and more!
- Close your eyes.
- For just a few minutes, breathe in and out, focusing on each breath.

- When your mind starts to wander (it will), gently and without judgment, bring your attention back to your breath.
- A good trick is to count seconds as you breathe (breathe in for 5 seconds, hold it for 5 seconds, breathe out for 5 seconds, hold it for 5 seconds, etc.).
- When you're ready, open your eyes and observe how you feel (there is no right or wrong answer to this!).

In the Breath of Life box, jot down your current mood and how long you spent doing your deep breathing practice. It's likely you will have great ideas while taking your deep breaths, so keep a notepad nearby (or use the reflection section of your journal) in case you want to scribble them down after you're done. This is a practice you can do any time throughout your day for mega benefits, beyond your journaling practice.

Sweet-Ass Affirmations

I am...

Because you are reading this, you're already thinking about ways to become a better version of you. Earlier, while you were setting your 100-day visions/goals, we discussed the power of affirming your visions in the present tense. There is a universal law we are quite fond of and would love to share: positive thoughts will breed more positivity in your life, and negative thoughts will breed more negativity in your life. Being a glass half full person will do wonders on its own, but what if we told you that you can become anyone and experience anything you want if you only think about these visions in the present tense, and then take action to support your vision?

Most of us grow up unaware of this power, and we tend to think about our current situation and our future based on the ideas of how society thinks we should be. Before we know it, we feel unhappy, lost, and out of touch with our dreams and visions. We may even find ourselves face-down-pants-down in the bushes next to a bottle of empty hooch.

The only thing you *must* do to become the person you dream of is to think about becoming that person, and then make a commitment to move in that direction. If you truly believe the transformation you desire will come true, and you commit your most valuable daily actions (which we will cover next) to work in unison with your beliefs, you will manifest the life of your dreams.

We are not implying that if you think of what you want, it will just magically appear without you doing anything. You must commit. Traditional woo-woo affirmation practices may lead you to believe that you can just sit in your room and repeat "I am a skinny and fit millionaire" and it will come true. It will **never** come true if you sit on your couch every day slaying buckets of fried chicken and episodes of Jerry Springer without making any commitment to bring it to life, no matter how many times you repeat it. You cannot bring an affirmation to life unless you are committed to it with your mind and actions.

If you ask the universe for water, it will quench your thirst. If you support your vision with all your energy, your vision will come to pass. Whatever you are reaching for, in return, is reaching for you! You are the sculptor of your own life.

"We become what we think about." - Earl Nightingale

There is an old speech from Earl Nightingale called *The Strangest Secret* that will blow your mind on the topic of manifesting visions. Before you continue this journal, please take a moment to listen to this 30-minute speech, seriously. We promise it will change your life. Don't be a donkey.

You can listen to this speech and gain access to all the other free bonus material mentioned in this journal by visiting: **www.sweetassjournal.com/pladbonus**

Earl argues that we become what we think about. The thoughts we have about our lives directly determine the outcome of our lives. Each one of us is the sum total of our thoughts, and by thinking we are great, we will become great.

This is not a new concept. Napoleon Hill's *Think and Grow Rich* expanded upon it, and so have other mass publications. It would be nearly impossible to go through the 100+ creative entrepreneur interviews Heath conducted and find someone who didn't affirm their future to transform into the person they are today. In one conversation with Bri Seeley, serial entrepreneur and author of *Permission to Leap*, she elaborated on a morning routine in which she and a few accountability friends had phone conversations where they addressed their future lives in the present tense.

They had conversations as their future selves, talking about how awesome their lives were and all the incredible things they were involved in (even though they weren't a reality yet). By doing this, they planted the seeds for their visions to manifest. (As you sow, so shall you reap.)

Philosophers, religious leaders, and successful people since the history of documented literature have used the power of visualization to manifest desired outcomes in life.

Now it's your turn.

What do you want in life?

Take a moment right now to think about what you truly want in life. What kind of person will you be, and what kind of lifestyle will you have if you are living with optimal happiness and health?

- What do you want to accomplish in your short time on this beautiful planet?
- What do you want to accomplish in this moment? In your love life? In your career?
- What areas in your life do you want to improve, like your relationships, your health, or your financial status?
- Do you have emotional pain points that need healing?
- Where do you want to live and travel?
- What have you always wanted to do more than anything in the world?
- What new skill sets would you like to learn?
- What would make your experience on Earth more meaningful?
- What internal areas do you want to develop the most? Self-image, confidence, honesty, bravery, respect?
- How many resistance gremlins do you want to body-slam today?
- What would it feel like to have full control of your diabetic journey, resulting in optimal happiness and health?

How do the answers to these questions relate to the visions that you set at the beginning of this journal? Remember, whatever it is you want, you can and will have it if you set an intention and take action toward it every day. By thinking about it, you will prime your brain to influence your behavior and decisions in favor of your visions, and you will become what you think about.

To create your sweet-ass affirmations, write your visions and desires in the present tense, then repeat them out loud three times each. If you want to get a little fancier, add an action to the end of the affirmation that supports how you will achieve the affirmation.

For example: I am the healthiest I have ever been **because I monitor my diet and exercise routine daily.**

This extra step will program both your conscious and subconscious mind to focus on the results you desire.

We have been on both sides of the fence ourselves. Before using affirmations, success was hard to pinpoint in our lives, careers, and creative projects. We struggled to identify the direction we were moving in, and we were also slaves to the walk-in closets full of emotional baggage that we were hiding from. We started by answering all the questions above, and then began writing our affirmations and reading them out loud daily.

This journal is a prime example of one of the many affirmation manifestations that once started as a simple sentence on a piece of paper.

"I have created a sweet-ass journal to help diabetics optimize their lifestyle."

The sentence was true long before the journal birthed into the physical world because we took daily action to make it happen.

Here are a few examples to give you ideas of what to write:

- I have a healthy relationship with my diabetes and give it the respect it requires.
- I make $100 extra per month on my side business.
- I am diabetes complications-free.
- I am confident and excited when I speak in public because I have nothing to fear.
- I am happy with my A1c and time in range.
- I save $200 a week by being aware of my spending, and I use it to pay off my debt.
- I am so happy and grateful for each moment of my life.
- I am focused on my vision, and nothing can stop me.
- I have an amazing support system that I can reach out to/lean on when I need to.
- I am in a healthy, fruitful relationship with Abundance.
- I create and sell my own products that help people discover happiness.
- I wake up at 5:00 every morning to meditate, read, write, and practice my guitar.
- I am happy, healthy and full of clarity because I decide to be.
- I write 500 words per day before I go to work.
- I have $10,000 in my bank account.
- I am the healthiest I have ever been because I monitor my diet and exercise routine daily.

- I am pain-free and my body feels incredible.
- I am in the best relationship possible and we constantly honor love, growth, and communication.
- I am confident in my abilities to live the longest, fullest, and best life I can.

Affirmations can be specific to a goal, but they can also be specific to an emotional pattern or thought.

If you want additional ideas for affirmations, check out **Sweet-Ass Affirmations: Motivation for Your Creative Maniac Mind** (Available on Ragecreate.com and Amazon.com).

It's your turn! In the Sweet-Ass Affirmations sections which appear in both the AM and PM, write out your affirmations and repeat them out loud. Start with a few simple affirmations, and you will naturally work your way into the miracle stages. When you read them, visualize them playing like a movie in your head at the same time. If you can do this simple practice, you will juice your brain to focus on becoming this new sweet-ass version of you, and your decisions and behavior will start to bring your visions to the present tense. Make the commitment to link your most valuable daily actions (next section) to your affirmations, and you will become what you think about.

This is a phenomenal habit to juice early upon waking and just before sleepy time!

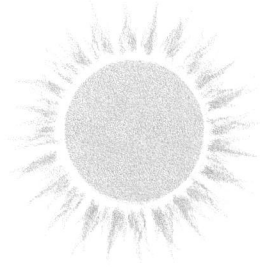

MORNING SECTIONS
GUIDE

Most-Valuable Daily Actions

What are the two most valuable actions I will take today to progress toward my goals, dreams, and optimal health?

By this point, you have already set your three sweet-ass visions for these 100 days of journaling. The next step is taking daily actions that prioritize your visions over all other to-do list mumbo jumbo. We use the word "actions" instead of "tasks" because "tasks" feels like a bad word. A task feels like a burden, and working toward optimal health and happiness is NOT a burden. It's a rollercoaster of miraculous action, and we *love* action because it's exciting!

It's no secret that being a goal-oriented person will greatly increase your ability to live a productive and accomplished life. If you're like us, though, sometimes having goals seems overwhelming. Just as we used to do, instead of setting goals and working toward them, you may opt for not setting them at all because it's easier and more comfortable. There is nothing to fall short of, so there is nothing to fear, right? No! This poopoo mindset will leave you wallowing in the mundane ocean far away from your potential, never to experience the magic of how it feels to build and sustain your own optimal lifestyle! The only thing you need to set goals and achieve them is motivation and action. You already have the motivation, or you wouldn't be reading this. You have already set your goals, so you are on a rampage already! So how do you implement the action *every day* to bring these goals to life?

Make your goals a priority over all other things that 'need' to be done. It seems so obvious, but it's something we all overlook. **What we do in the short term, in the moment, is the seed for everything we will manifest in the future.** You don't need any more motivation, you just need to break your habit of hesitation and take action. The more action you take in the short term to work on something long term, the faster it comes to life. If you work on your Spanish for 20 minutes each month, then it will most likely take decades before you know the basics of Spanish. If you work on your Spanish for 20 minutes each day over a 100-day period, you'll be speaking basic Spanish within 100 days! Twenty minutes per day over 100 days is 33.33 hours of Spanish—the near equivalent of a semester course.

Creating a daily habit to work on what is *most important* over all other to-do list items is the key to bringing your vision to reality. Heath had the pleasure of interviewing multiple international, NY Times, and Amazon best-selling authors, including the lovely Honorée Corder who has sold over 800,000 copies of her books including Vision to Reality, Prosperity for Writers, and You Must Write a Book. If you ask Honorée about the key to her writing success, she will tell you that it all starts with simply writing **every day**, over anything else. She lets nothing stand in the way of her daily writing habit. Thus nothing can stop her from achieving her goals (like selling 800,000 books).

If your goal is to create the healthiest version of your mind and body, then gear your daily actions toward body movement, stretching, meal management, meditation, and water intake.

If your goal is to reduce your A1c and maintain it, then gear your daily actions toward testing more, taking all your medications, or finding a meal plan you really enjoy which does not cause major fluctuations in your blood sugars.

If your goal is to pay off personal debt, then gear your daily actions toward financial restructuring, like eliminating unnecessary bills, creating an aggressive savings plan, or simply spending $10 less at the grocery store that day.

If your goal is to write a novel about your crazy high-school English teacher who used to try to sell you weed, then gear your daily actions toward writing 200 words per day, designing your cover, or brainstorming a marketing plan.

When you picked up this journal, you planted the seeds for manifesting your success. Whatever you are working toward (your sweet-ass visions), literally picture them as the bud of a flower. To get from the seeds to the buds, you must supply the energy needed to grow the stems! Your daily actions will grow into beautiful buds if you supply them with your essential energy. If you use your essential energy on other things like social media rabbit holes or watching people get spray tans on reality television, there won't be any energy for your buds to bloom.

Set your most valuable daily actions in direct relation to the sweet-ass visions you are working toward, and use your best energy to complete these actions before all other things. If you can do this every day, you will blow the top off your campaign for optimal happiness, health, and lifestyle.

Big Cheese

What makes me smile and why?

To create a life of happiness is to fill life with smiles. By definition, a smile is "a pleased, kind, or amused facial expression." If smiles are the result of pleasure, kindness, amusement, and excitement, then a natural smile is a building block of long-term happiness. To increase our smiles, we must build our awareness of people, places, and things that bring us pleasure, kindness, amusement, and excitement. We must regularly pause and identify these things that make us happy and the things that we are grateful for. What easier way than taking a moment, every morning, to consider the root of our happiness and all parts of life we appreciate?

By making this our first step in the morning, we kickstart our magical day, setting a positive tone and energy. We paint pleasure, kindness, amusement, and excitement into all interactions and experiences throughout the rest of the day.

Have you ever woken up angry, knowing the job you despise or the chores you have to do lay in front of you? Because you flooded your mind with anger and discontent upon rising, you most likely felt bitter and unaware of all the beautiful things that make you happy. As you go about the rest of your day, you'll magnetically center on the negatives, resulting in an experience that is negative.

It works both ways!

You can reframe your mind to always think about happy things, filling the rest of your day with a happy mindset!

As soon as you start focusing on the pure joys that bring happiness to your life, everything begins to change. Because your awareness is now centered on positives, the negative resistance gremlins will get a kick in the ass out the door. Your brain is a magical beast that is a vital partner in your journey toward happiness and optimal living. This simple morning routine is the seed to a much larger and longer life of pure happiness and freedom.

Remember, there is no wrong way to fill out your boxes! Keep it short, jam-pack it full so it's running out of the box, or doodle something that makes you smile. Drawing rules too!

So, what makes you smile and why?

Examples of things that might make you smile:

> Significant others, family, kayaking, unicorns, flowers, being alive, sex, dancing, sports, donkeys, meditation, handwritten letters, colors, Jim Carrey, sweet mullets, sloths, professional wrestling outfits, places with carb counts, nature, the stars, scuba diving, giving gifts, level blood sugars, practical jokes, world travel, getting an awesome A1c, streaking, cartoons, supplies being covered by insurance, skydiving, accomplishing goals, successfully trying new recipes, fist-pumping, people watching at Grateful Dead concerts, Danny DeVito, free samples, connecting with new friends, a Friday night cocktail, working in your undies, a hot bath, creating something, snowboarding, finishing a hard workout, giving compliments, receiving compliments, food trucks, beaches, and giving wedgies to resistance gremlins.

In addition, make sure you write down *why* they make you smile. This pulls the value from the object in your life to the front and identifies the gratitude within. Start your mornings by thinking about what makes you smile, and your days will surely have a positive theme!

More on Gratitude

You can also look at this box as a space for practicing gratitude.

Sure, all the things that make you smile can also be things you're thankful for, but not everything you are thankful for necessarily makes you smile.

Practicing gratitude, or being thankful, is about pausing and appreciating yourself, all that surrounds you, and every interaction and experience of life. It's about focusing on the blessings we do have, as opposed to fixating on what we don't. It's easy to degrade ourselves because we aren't good looking enough, smart enough, or as wealthy as others we know. But degrading yourself is just a mental version of soiling on yourself, and nobody wants to experience that (except one dude we know).

A simple daily act of logging all that you are thankful for, no matter how big or small, will help your mind focus on just how fortunate you are to be here now, just as you are. So many aspects of our lives seem invisible because we are never required to think about them, yet without them, our lives wouldn't be even close to the same. The focus of this section is to avoid taking anything for granted, and to build focus around the magical parts of life that hide in the dark and don't get enough credit (and no, we are not talking about your rock-solid booty). Pack out this box with anything and everything you are thankful for. It helps to elaborate on why you're thankful for them, too.

Sweet-Ass Reward

Although plenty of rewards will show up in your life while you practice the habits within this journal over 100 days, sometimes it will feel like you are working your ass off, especially with your valuable daily actions.

While long-term rewards and benefits are amazing, you also deserve to enjoy the ride on a daily basis in celebration of your commitment, actions, and effort.

Toward the end of each morning practice, you will see the Sweet-Ass Reward section. In this space, choose a reward to give yourself after you accomplish your two most valuable daily actions. Party!!!

Yeah, eating a tub of ice cream every day isn't exactly healthy, but rewarding yourself with a bowl once a week for accomplishing your actions makes it extra sweet! Or, perhaps, you can take yourself out to get a nice massage or dinner to celebrate your progress.

Some days your rewards will be massively exciting, and other days they might be small and humble. Either way, make sure you are taking care of yourself and enjoying the ride. Buy yourself some flowers. Go see that movie! Spend a night out with your friends! Read a good book for an hour in the bath! To develop ultimate levels of happiness, it's important to surround yourself with exciting people and activities that you truly enjoy. The rewards box is an incredible way to work those into your journey!

Wildcard Box

Wanna keep things exciting? The last box in the AM section of the journal is the Wildcard Box. Every day, the contents of this box will change. Sometimes the wildcard will present simple facts and thoughts, and other times it will introduce new systems for developing happiness and optimizing your lifestyle.

We won't reveal all the goodies the box will share with you, but instead we'll leave it a mystery of excitement for your 100-day journey!

The further you wander into your journey, the more value you will uncover!

Are you ready? :)

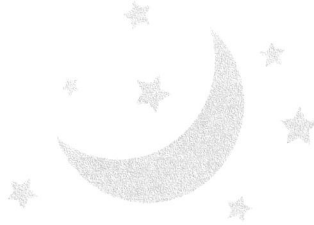

EVENING SECTIONS
GUIDE

Winning

My wins for the day are...

We have mentioned the importance of paying attention to the positive side of life. Plant positive seeds and grow positive vines. What better way to keep the motivation rocket flying at full speed than to celebrate the wins that fuel your rocket as it blasts through space?

This section is simple: write down everything you do throughout the day *except* for negative things that hinder your progress. We do not want you to focus on the negatives because most of the time they poison your mindset and attract more negativity. However, problems or negative situations that do arise always have an underlying opportunity for positive change. If you can identify the opportunity, it's totally acceptable to include the opportunity as a win in this section as well.

When we say write down everything, we mean *everything*. The point of this section is to show you just how much you actually do accomplish in a single day. It's mind-boggling once you start writing down all the little and big wins you accomplish. Not only will it remind you of your brilliant capabilities, but it will also highlight the time throughout the day that you may often take for granted.

When you do this practice, you'll start paying attention to the beauty in all things, big and small. You will start to appreciate the 10 minutes alone you had with your significant other in the midst of a hectic day. You will start to cherish parts of life we rarely even think about, like our ability to wake up every morning, see the love around us, and use our magical hands and brains to bring creations into the world. You will start to understand that life is full of wins in each moment we experience. We are winning because we are writing this right now. You are winning because you are reading it. We are winning because we are alive, and breathing, and experiencing this world with all our senses. Everything is in its right place.

So before you lay your pretty little head down on your pillow, haystack, or giant furry pup at night (sorry cat people), start your PM practice by writing down your WINS for the day. Don't just write the big things. Write anything and everything you do that contributes to your moving forward! Waking up is a gift! Eating your meals is a gift! Returning safely from work is a gift! As you continue this practice, you'll start to notice something incredible: Your wins will get bigger and more powerful. You will build a massive awareness of all you accomplish, which will become a huge motivator to keep dominating.

Here are a few things we have used in our wins list to help you brainstorm some ideas:

- Had a full and restorative night's sleep with no interruptions
- Meditated for 10 minutes on abundance and gratitude
- Wrote two new blogs on how to beat diabetes burnout
- Listened to my favorite artists while dancing and cooking dinner
- Blood sugar was "in range" 85% of the day
- Woke up breathing in my warm, cozy bed
- Washed my face, brushed my teeth, used my homemade mouthwash
- Woke up with a beautiful BG of 90
- Filled out my sweet-ass journal morning section and meditated for 5 minutes
- Found a new low-carb ice cream which is actually delicious!!
- Walked outside barefoot and looked at the stars before the sun came up
- Enjoyed a hot green tea while reading The War of Art
- Received a text from an old friend that I hadn't spoken to in awhile
- Drank a hot cup of Hawaiian coffee while wrapped in a fuzzy blanket
- Went on a mile jog with my pup and did some pushups
- Brainstormed a new creative project for my website
- Fixed the motor inducer in the heater
- Brainstormed with Dad about a new invention
- Mapped out a delicious meal plan
- Created a new bills and budget spreadsheet to help manage cash flow and eliminate debt
- Stopped to smell the roses outside my front door before going to a coffee shop to work
- Started a fun minimalist game to get rid of all the junk I own that isn't valuable to my journey
- Spent awesome quality time with the family
- Created a very rough sketch of how a podcast flows for podcasting business idea
- Watched my fish tank for 20 calming minutes

- Paid for a stranger's coffee just to see them smile
- Called my grandma
- Rewarded myself with a new book after finishing my daily actions
- Folded all my laundry and cleaned the kitchen
- Watched a cool documentary about plant medicine on YouTube
- Have started filling out the PM section of this journal

Now it's your turn to create the magic. Each day is a mini battle in your war against resistance gremlins, and each win you have throughout the day is a blow to the heart of those slimy little bastards. Every night, dedicate a few minutes to write down all your wins! Alternatively, keep a small journal or notecard in your pocket to write them down as they occur throughout the day, and then glue them to your journal or write them in. Hot glue guns are all the rage! Start the streak. Keep winning the battles. Defeat the fear and resistance gremlins. Conquer your optimal lifestyle!

Party Checklist

To party like a diabetic, you gotta keep a party list handy at all times. If you want to feel your best as often as possible, you have to keep track of items you are carrying around in your party pants that contribute to the happiest, healthiest version of you.

We created the Party Checklist to help remind you of certain tools throughout your journey that are vital for your optimal well-being.

Here is a brief overview of the items that will appear in the checklist:

Rx
Whether you are taking injectable, inhalable, or oral medications, it is important to do so consistently. If you are on multiple medications throughout the day, consider putting an alarm on your phone or computer to help remind you or pair it with an action you do every day (such as brushing your teeth, showering, eating lunch, etc). If you don't take medications daily, don't worry about checking this off!

Test
Checking your blood glucose helps you know how certain foods, actions, and stressors affect you. It also helps you stay safe from going too low (hypoglycemia) or too high (hyperglycemia). Remember, your levels are not a report card—simply a number to help you make choices! Be sure to test as often as your doctor recommends, and check this party box when applicable.

Water Intake
We all know how important it is to drink water, but as a person with diabetes, it is crucial for you to stay hydrated. Dehydration can cause stubborn or increased blood sugars. We recommend you drink two liters throughout the day, and more if it is hot out! Double points if you check this off while sipping on some H2O.

Reward
Check the reward box in the PM section of your journal to verify that you rewarded yourself for completing your most valuable daily actions. You don't have to reward yourself every day, but it's a good practice to treat yourself to something nice as often as possible, especially when you are making amazing progress.

Nutrition & Movement (introduced later)
Nutrition and movement are both vital parts of creating your optimal diabetic lifestyle. We will guide you through these processes later in the journal, and once we do, you'll want to check the corresponding boxes in the PM to verify you're sticking to your goals and keeping your healthy streaks alive.

At the end of each day, when you are doodling your amazing progress into the evening section of the journal, make sure to fill out your party checklist. The dance floor is waiting for your disco moves.

Planning Ahead: Tomorrow's Most Valuable Daily Actions

What are the two most valuable actions I will take tomorrow to progress toward my goals, dreams, and optimal health?

Just as you set your daily actions for the day, it's just as important to plan the following day's actions at night. By setting your intentions to dominate the following day before you go to sleep, you prepare your brain for success the next day.

Nighttime is the perfect opportunity to reflect on your progress for the day, allowing you to easily focus on the next important step in your journey to grow and bloom your sweet-ass freedom buds. You won't lay in bed thinking about all the possible things you may have to do tomorrow. Instead, you will accomplish a state of relaxation, and your body and mind will get the rest they need to become your war tanks of efficiency and effectiveness in your daily battles against the gremlins.

You will subconsciously encourage yourself to wake up earlier because you have a purpose for the day. Because you have a purpose, you will be in a much stronger position to judo-chop the procrastination gremlins in the throat before they can attempt to haunt your thoughts.

Every day we are faced with multiple decisions and unique problem-solving scenarios, so setting our intentions the night before will help reserve the willpower we need for other parts of life throughout the day.

Yes, it may seem redundant writing your freedom actions the night before AND the morning of your rampage, but think of it as an opportunity for extra preparation. When you are more prepared, you are more likely to feel motivated and confident, and you will position yourself for success.

Remember to focus on the two most important actions for the following day (as discussed in the AM daily actions section) and to attack the scariest and hairiest first! When you accomplish the action you most fear before anything else, the rest of the day is like busting into the secret levels in a video game. Everything becomes a bonus round!

Reflection and Thoughts

How awesome was today? How challenging was today? How are you feeling? What are you thinking about? How did it feel to complete your daily actions? What were your thoughts during your deep breathing sessions? What are you currently observing about your world? What trends did you notice with your blood sugars?

This section helps you reflect upon the awesomeness and hardship you experience throughout the day. It's a final check-in before you head to rest that pretty little face! There are no exact guidelines on how to use this box. It's 100% free for you to do your own thing! If you want to staple a picture of Ryan Gosling to it, we are sure nobody will complain.

As a human, you will naturally go through periods of streaks and droughts. It happens to all of us. The most important thing is to stay on track with creating the habit, and giving 111% effort whenever possible to maximize your awakening into the optimal lifestyle that you are creating. Don't be hard on yourself. Instead, be proud of what you do accomplish. You kick supreme ass.

Are you ready to make magic?

PART 3:
THE JOURNAL

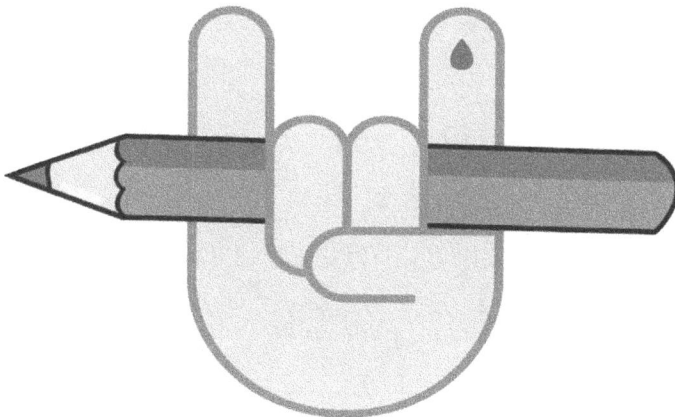

Time to Party and Never Give Up

Because your happiness, health, and lifestyle are worth it...

It's not easy having diabetes. There are so many factors that go into managing this disease and at times it can just suck. This journal is *not* intended to overwhelm you or cause you stress and anxiety. If it does, just like with deep breathing, you are the exact type of person that should be using it! It's so easy from a fearful and unhappy place to let resistance cripple us. It can be a real struggle to read books, journal, or simply reflect on our lives when we are suffocating with fear. This dark space can end up convincing us to ignore our dreams and efforts for self-improvement in exchange for the big illusionary comfort blanket full of quick and shallow stimulation and distraction. Being comfortable is easier than creating habits to support your optimal lifestyle, but there is no growth in comfort. Everything you have ever dreamed of is sleeping on the other side of your comfort zone. Think of this journal as your secret weapon to defeat the shadow armies of fear and resistance gremlins and fill it with energetic ammunition!

Even we, the creators of this journal, don't open the journal for weeks sometimes. Coincidently, those weeks are usually when we experience high stress, doubt, lack of confidence, and zero creativity. When we are on a roll and hitting three- or four-week streaks, everything seems to fall into place, and our creative drives are blessed with magical results and explosive opportunity. This journal has become an anchor for the creation of our optimal lifestyles, and as a result, the instigator of our sustainable happiness.

Do this for your health, your body, your happiness, and the person you deserve to become, no matter how big, small, briefly, or extensively you write. Take a step forward every day with this journal and create a habit to develop your optimal diabetic lifestyle. Your creative energy will flow into so many other areas of your life, and you will see color where it's always been gray. As the world is constantly "looking" for happiness everywhere and failing to find it, you will be one of the few who creates it yourself.

As Joseph Campbell teaches:

> "When you follow your bliss, that thing that truly electrifies you, four things automatically happen: you put yourself in the path of good luck, you meet the people you want to know, doors open where there weren't doors before, and doors open for you that wouldn't open to anybody else."

We hope this journal helps you discover your superpowers and optimize your bliss.

And, have a sweet-ass time along the way!

EXAMPLE OF COMPLETED JOURNAL

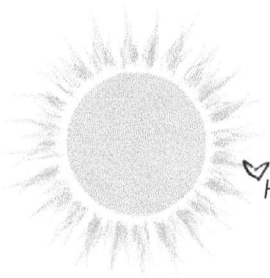

DATE ...11.... / ....19. / 20 .19...

Happiness is the absence of the striving for happiness.
– Chuang Tzu

BG: 87

Breath of Life

Close your eyes and breathe deeply for as long as possible.

Current Mood: Rested   Duration: 6 mins

Sweet-Ass Affirmations

debt free 💲💲

I am....

making a huge positive impact in the world ☺

injury and diabetes complication free

the healthiest I possibly can be in mind, body, and spirit

Confident in my decisions and actions

HAPPY

What are the two **most valuable actions** I will take today to progress toward my goals, dreams, and optimal health?

1. Schedule workouts for the rest of the week

2. Drink 2 more H₂O bottles than yesterday

What makes me ☺ and why?

good cup of coffee 1st thing in the morning
↳ makes me think of being @ home over holidays w/my parents

crisp autumn air
↳ refreshing & my fav season is here

Wildcard

Knowledge Bomb

Managing diabetes is not a science, it is an art.

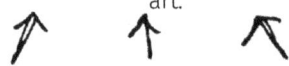

↑   ↑   ↖

Sweet-Ass Reward

How will I reward myself after accomplishing my two valuable actions today?

Setting aside 30 min to listen to my fav. relaxing music & a face mask

My **wins** for the day are:

signed on new PLAD partner
'in range' 92% of the day
(woot woot)
talked w/ mom & sis
dominated my workout
complimented a stranger
bought a bozuet of flowers
woke up rested !!

got free samples ☺

Party Checklist

☑ Rx ☑ Test ☑ Water ☐ Reward
½
↓
no face mask

Breath of Life

Close your eyes and breathe deeply for as long as possible.

Current Mood: grounded   Duration: 9.5 mins

What are the two **most valuable actions** I will take tomorrow to progress toward my goals, dreams, and optimal health?

1. Create schedule for upcoming trip

2. Stick to meal plan (AKA dont skip lunch)

Sweet-Ass Affirmations

living my best life   I am.... happy & healthy ✓ ☺ ♡

injury & diabetes $[debt free]$
complication free

the healthiest I possibly can be   in a fun, loving, and
in mind, body, and spirit   committed relationship
w/ my best friend
making a HUGE and positive impact on the world

Reflection and Thoughts

I finally allowed myself to just relax and be today.
I have been pushing for so long that I didn't realize how
tired I was! It was nice to sit back & realize that
I could still be productive w/o being high strung (pretty
sure the cat appreciated it too...)

You are   1% done with optimizing your diabetic lifestyle. ☺   BG: 121

OPTIMIZE YOUR DIABETIC LIFESTYLE IN 100 DAYS

Please visit the following link to **download all the bonus material** mentioned throughout this journal, including a **free 100-day checklist** you can print and put on your wall to remind you to keep your journal streak rolling!

www.sweetassjournal.com/pladbonus

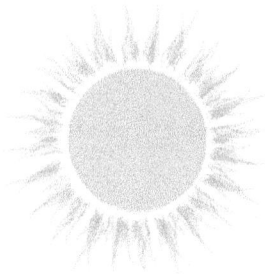

DATE .... / .... / 20 ....

Happiness is the absence of the striving for happiness.
– Chuang Tzu

BG:

Breath of Life

Close your eyes and breathe deeply for as long as possible.

Current Mood: Duration:

Sweet-Ass Affirmations

I am....

What are the two **most valuable actions** I will take today to progress toward my goals, dreams, and optimal health?

1.

2.

What makes me ☺ and why?

Wildcard

Knowledge Bomb

Managing diabetes is not a science, it is an art.

Sweet-Ass Reward

How will I reward myself after accomplishing my two valuable actions today?

My **wins** for the day are:

Party Checklist

☐ Rx ☐ Test ☐ Water ☐ Reward

Breath of Life

Close your eyes and breathe deeply for as long as possible.

Current Mood: Duration:

What are the two **most valuable actions** I will take tomorrow to progress toward my goals, dreams, and optimal health?

1.

2.

Sweet-Ass Affirmations

I am....

Reflection and Thoughts

You are   **1**% done with optimizing your diabetic lifestyle. ☺   **BG:**

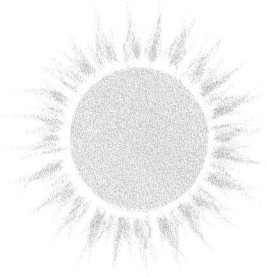

DATE .... / .... / 20 ....

Start making decisions based on who you want to be,
not on who you are right now.
– Amber Ludwig-Vilhauer

BG:

Breath of Life

Close your eyes and breathe deeply for as long as possible.

Current Mood: Duration:

Sweet-Ass Affirmations

I am....

What are the two **most valuable actions** I will take today to progress toward my goals, dreams, and optimal health?

1.

2.

What makes me ☺ and why?

Wildcard

Knowledge Bomb

Testing your blood sugar is a learning experience, not a report card.

Sweet-Ass Reward

How will I reward myself after accomplishing my two valuable actions today?

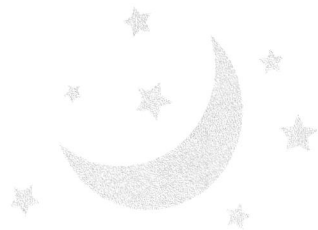

My **wins** for the day are:

Party Checklist

☐ Rx ☐ Test ☐ Water ☐ Reward

Breath of Life

Close your eyes and breathe deeply for as long as possible.

Current Mood: Duration:

What are the two **most valuable actions** I will take tomorrow to
progress toward my goals, dreams, and optimal health?

1.

2.

Sweet-Ass Affirmations

I am....

Reflection and Thoughts

You are   2 % done with optimizing your diabetic lifestyle. ☺   **BG:**

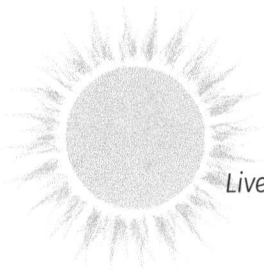

DATE .... / .... / 20 ....

Live the life you have while you create the life of your dreams.
– Hal Elrod

BG:

Breath of Life

Close your eyes and breathe deeply for as long as possible.

Current Mood: Duration:

Sweet-Ass Affirmations

I am....

What are the two **most valuable actions** I will take today to progress toward my goals, dreams, and optimal health?

1.

2.

What makes me ☺ and why?

Wildcard

Knowledge Bomb

A good night's sleep helps improve and stabilize blood sugars.

Sweet-Ass Reward

How will I reward myself after accomplishing my two valuable actions today?

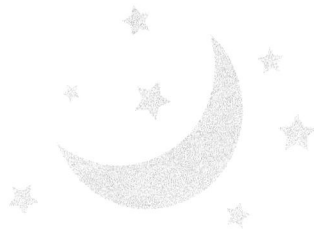

My **wins** for the day are:

Party Checklist

☐ Rx ☐ Test ☐ Water ☐ Reward

Breath of Life

Close your eyes and breathe deeply for as long as possible.

Current Mood: Duration:

What are the two **most valuable actions** I will take tomorrow to progress toward my goals, dreams, and optimal health?

1.

2.

Sweet-Ass Affirmations

I am....

Reflection and Thoughts

You are **3** % done with optimizing your diabetic lifestyle. ☺

BG:

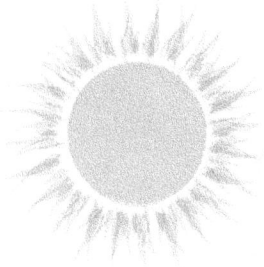

DATE .... / .... / 20 ....

The more you find good in the other, the more you find good in yourself, no matter what the other is.
– Mike Dooley

BG:

Breath of Life

Close your eyes and breathe deeply for as long as possible.

Current Mood: Duration:

Sweet-Ass Affirmations

I am....

What are the two **most valuable actions** I will take today to progress toward my goals, dreams, and optimal health?

1.

2.

What makes me ☺ and why?

Wildcard

Knowledge Bomb

Stress can make blood sugars harder to manage due to hormones such as adrenaline and cortisol.

Sweet-Ass Reward

How will I reward myself after accomplishing my two valuable actions today?

My **wins** for the day are:

Party Checklist

☐ Rx   ☐ Test   ☐ Water   ☐ Reward

Breath of Life

Close your eyes and breathe deeply for as long as possible.

Current Mood: Duration:

What are the two **most valuable actions** I will take tomorrow to
progress toward my goals, dreams, and optimal health?

1.

2.

Sweet-Ass Affirmations

I am....

Reflection and Thoughts

You are   4 % done with optimizing your diabetic lifestyle. ☺

BG:

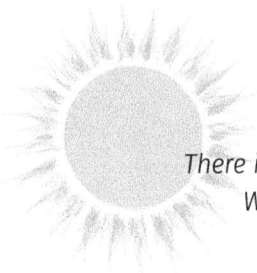

DATE .... / .... / 20 ....

There is nothing so wretched or foolish as to anticipate misfortunes.
What madness it is in your expecting evil before it arrives!
– Seneca

BG:

Breath of Life

Close your eyes and breathe deeply for as long as possible.

Current Mood: Duration:

Sweet-Ass Affirmations

I am....

What are the two **most valuable actions** I will take today to progress toward my goals, dreams, and optimal health?

1.

2.

What makes me ☺ and why?

Sweet-Ass Reward

How will I reward myself after accomplishing my two valuable actions today?

Wildcard

Meditation Resources

A few cool apps to get you started with deeper breathing and meditation:

Insight Meditation Timer
Headspace
Calm

(Links available at
www.sweetassjournal.com/pladbonus)

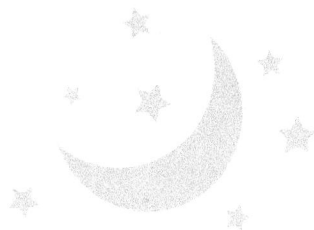

My **wins** for the day are:

Party Checklist

☐ Rx   ☐ Test   ☐ Water   ☐ Reward

Breath of Life

Close your eyes and breathe deeply for as long as possible.

Current Mood: Duration:

What are the two **most valuable actions** I will take tomorrow to
progress toward my goals, dreams, and optimal health?

1.

2.

Sweet-Ass Affirmations

I am....

Reflection and Thoughts

You are   5 % done with optimizing your diabetic lifestyle. ☺   **BG:**

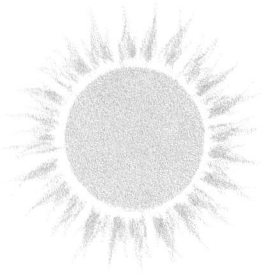

DATE .... / .... / 20 ....

It is not enough to be busy. So are the ants.
The question is: What are we busy about?
– Henry David Thoreau

BG:

Breath of Life

Close your eyes and breathe deeply for as long as possible.

Current Mood: Duration:

Sweet-Ass Affirmations

I am....

What are the two **most valuable actions** I will take today to progress toward my goals, dreams, and optimal health?

1.

2.

What makes me ☺ and why?

Wildcard

Break Dance

Give yourself a break! Set aside time in your day to do something you really love (like dancing).

Sweet-Ass Reward

How will I reward myself after accomplishing my two valuable actions today?

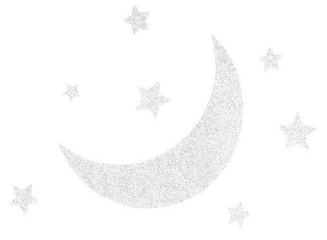

My **wins** for the day are:

Party Checklist

☐ Rx ☐ Test ☐ Water ☐ Reward

Breath of Life

Close your eyes and breathe deeply for as long as possible.

Current Mood: Duration:

What are the two **most valuable actions** I will take tomorrow to
progress toward my goals, dreams, and optimal health?

1.

2.

Sweet-Ass Affirmations

I am....

Reflection and Thoughts

You are   **6** % done with optimizing your diabetic lifestyle. ☺   **BG:**

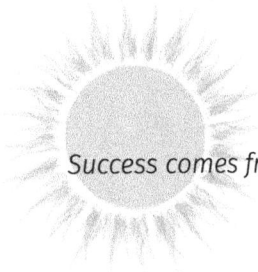

DATE .... / .... / 20 ....

Success comes from good judgment. Good judgment depends mostly on experience, and experience usually comes from poor judgment.
– Unknown

BG:

Breath of Life

Close your eyes and breathe deeply for as long as possible.

Current Mood: Duration:

Sweet-Ass Affirmations

I am....

What are the two **most valuable actions** I will take today to progress toward my goals, dreams, and optimal health?

1.

2.

What makes me ☺ and why?

Wildcard

Knowledge Bomb

Be careful how you speak to yourself, because you are listening.

Sweet-Ass Reward

How will I reward myself after accomplishing my two valuable actions today?

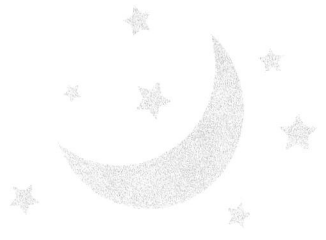

My **wins** for the day are:

Party Checklist

☐ Rx   ☐ Test   ☐ Water   ☐ Reward

Breath of Life

Close your eyes and breathe deeply for as long as possible.

Current Mood: Duration:

What are the two **most valuable actions** I will take tomorrow to progress toward my goals, dreams, and optimal health?

1.

2.

Sweet-Ass Affirmations

I am....

Reflection and Thoughts

You are   **7** % done with optimizing your diabetic lifestyle. ☺

BG:

Wildcard: Exercise and Movement — Show that Beautiful Body Some Love

Whether you like to take long walks on the beach, do chores around the house, or win triathlons, movement and exercise are incredibly helpful in managing diabetes. By moving your body, you are signaling your muscles to take up more glucose from the bloodstream, which ultimately could lower blood sugar levels. Movement and exercise also help the body become more sensitive to insulin (therefore reducing insulin resistance) so it can do its job more effectively.

The type of activity you do could affect your levels differently. Moderate aerobic activity, such as walking, stretching, easy bike rides, etc., typically lower glucose levels. More intense or anaerobic movement such as heavy weight lifting, sprints, or cage fighting a bear can increase levels due to stress hormones. Depending on how your body reacts to movement, it is important to keep tabs on your glucose levels and have fast-acting glucose available just in case it decides to drop it like its hot.

Here are a few movement ideas for you to either start or to add to your routine:
- Dance class
- Group fitness
- Run/walk in the park with your dog
- Take the stairs instead of the escalator or elevator
- Suggest a walking meeting
- Crossfit
- Yoga
- Barre
- Pilates
- Bodyweight exercises such as squats, push-ups, sit-ups, etc. that don't require equipment
- High-intensity interval training (HIIT) or Tabata
- Kickboxing
- Hiking
- Mountain biking
- Ice climbing

Make sure to check out the bonus materials for a ton more ideas and videos on how to incorporate more activity into your life.

Heads up that from now on, movement will be added to the party checklist. So after getting your sweat (we prefer glisten) on, make sure to check it off.

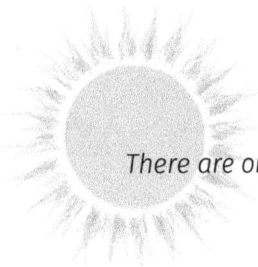

DATE .... / .... / 20 ....

There are only two ways to live your life. One is as though nothing is a miracle.
The other is as though everything is a miracle.
– Albert Einstein

BG:

Breath of Life

Close your eyes and breathe deeply for as long as possible.

Current Mood: Duration:

Sweet-Ass Affirmations

I am....

What are the two **most valuable actions** I will take today to progress toward my goals, dreams, and optimal health?

1.

2.

What makes me ☺ and why?

Wildcard

Exercise / Movement

Have you moved that sexy body yet today? Choose a few exercises on your own or from the bonus material and get that blood flowing!

Sweet-Ass Reward

How will I reward myself after accomplishing my two valuable actions today?

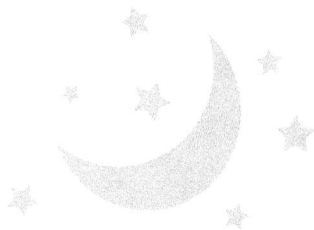

My **wins** for the day are:

Party Checklist

☐ Rx   ☐ Test   ☐ Water

☐ Movement   ☐ Reward

Breath of Life

Close your eyes and breathe deeply for as long as possible.

Current Mood: Duration:

What are the two **most valuable actions** I will take tomorrow to progress toward my goals, dreams, and optimal health?

1.

2.

Sweet-Ass Affirmations

I am....

Reflection and Thoughts

You are   8 % done with optimizing your diabetic lifestyle. ☺

BG:

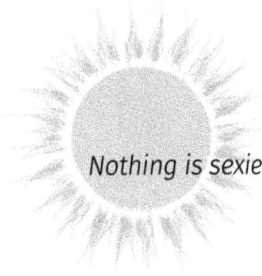

DATE .... / .... / 20 ....

Nothing is sexier than someone who is not afraid of being their true, authentic selves and honoring their spirit without the fear of being judged.
– Unknown

BG:

Breath of Life

Close your eyes and breathe deeply for as long as possible.

Current Mood: Duration:

Sweet-Ass Affirmations

I am....

What are the two **most valuable actions** I will take today to progress toward my goals, dreams, and optimal health?

1.

2.

What makes me ☺ and why?

Wildcard

Knowledge Bomb

Track your exercise and how it affects your blood sugar. Some activities may raise it, while others might lower it.

Sweet-Ass Reward

How will I reward myself after accomplishing my two valuable actions today?

My **wins** for the day are:

Party Checklist

☐ Rx ☐ Test ☐ Water

☐ Movement ☐ Reward

Breath of Life

Close your eyes and breathe deeply for as long as possible.

Current Mood: Duration:

What are the two **most valuable actions** I will take tomorrow to progress toward my goals, dreams, and optimal health?

1.

2.

Sweet-Ass Affirmations

I am....

Reflection and Thoughts

You are **9** % done with optimizing your diabetic lifestyle. ☺

BG:

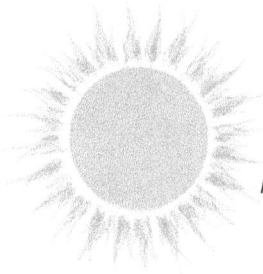

DATE .... / .... / 20 ....

Mindfulness leads to the discovery of your true essence.
– Molly Knight Forde

BG:

Breath of Life

Close your eyes and breathe deeply for as long as possible.

Current Mood: Duration:

Sweet-Ass Affirmations

I am....

What are the two **most valuable actions** I will take today to progress toward my goals, dreams, and optimal health?

1.

2.

What makes me ☺ and why?

Wildcard

Knowledge Bomb

During movement or exercise, the time of day can affect your blood sugar.

Sweet-Ass Reward

How will I reward myself after accomplishing my two valuable actions today?

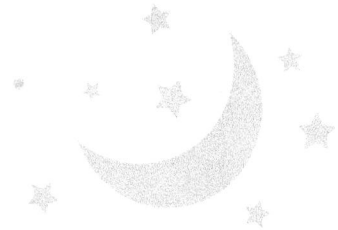

My **wins** for the day are:

Party Checklist

☐ Rx ☐ Test ☐ Water

☐ Movement ☐ Reward

Breath of Life

Close your eyes and breathe deeply for as long as possible.

Current Mood: Duration:

What are the two **most valuable actions** I will take tomorrow to progress toward my goals, dreams, and optimal health?

1.

2.

Sweet-Ass Affirmations

I am....

Reflection and Thoughts

Sweet-Ass Affirmations!

Occasionally, you will see affirmation cards appear between journaling days. These affirmations are paired with quick, witty motivational rants to explore the affirmation topic. May they bring you deep thoughts, giggles, and direction!

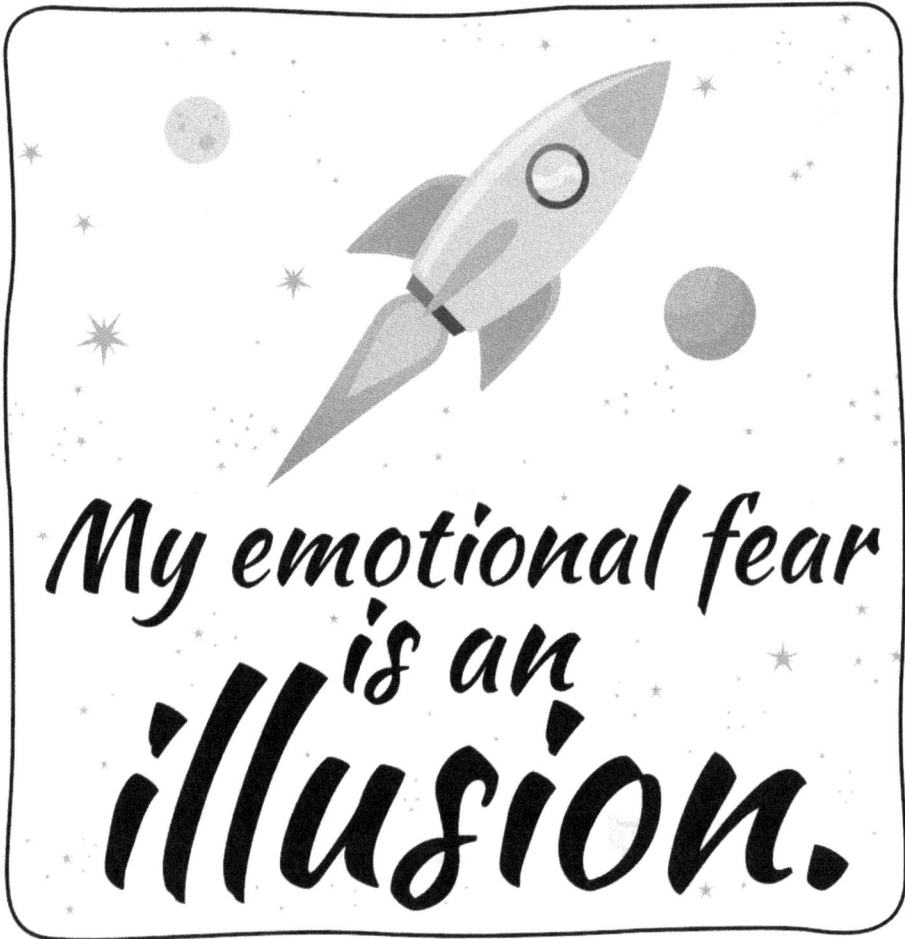

My emotional fear is an illusion.

You are a hunk of magical meat strapped to a skeleton made of stardust. You are raging through space on a giant rock at approximately 67,000 mph around a giant ball of fire in an infinite abyss. Be brave and bold in your quest, because you are a product of the impossible.

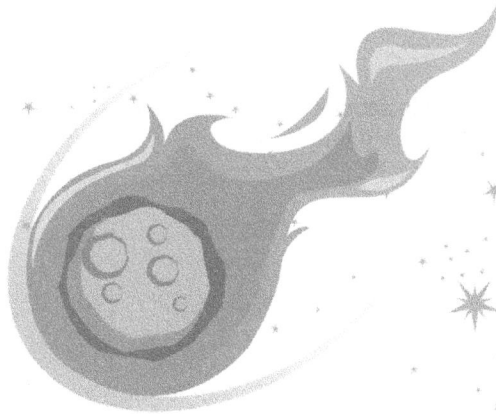

Rage Create

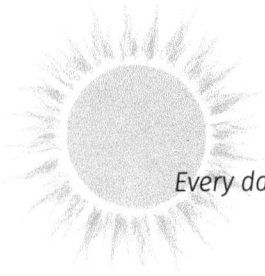

DATE .... / .... / 20 ....

Every day is a bonus round. Slow down and enjoy something beautiful.
– Sohrab Mirmont

BG:

Breath of Life

Close your eyes and breathe deeply for as long as possible.

Current Mood: Duration:

Sweet-Ass Affirmations

I am....

What are the two **most valuable actions** I will take today to progress toward my goals, dreams, and optimal health?

1.

2.

What makes me ☺ and why?

Wildcard

Knowledge Bomb

Exercise is a free drug; use it as much as possible!

Sweet-Ass Reward

How will I reward myself after accomplishing my two valuable actions today?

My **wins** for the day are:

Party Checklist

☐ Rx ☐ Test ☐ Water

☐ Movement ☐ Reward

Breath of Life

Close your eyes and breathe deeply for as long as possible.

Current Mood: Duration:

What are the two **most valuable actions** I will take tomorrow to progress toward my goals, dreams, and optimal health?

1.

2.

Sweet-Ass Affirmations

I am....

Reflection and Thoughts

You are **11**% done with optimizing your diabetic lifestyle. ☺

BG:

Wildcard: Creating Your Sacred Space

It's no secret that having a special space to create can throw a switch in your creative brain. Most students of creativity, meditation, and optimization will admit to receiving special inspiration from particular creative spaces that they revisit.

Without a structured plan, you may already find yourself returning to the same spot—a place where you think about or observe special areas of your life. By having a relaxed and peaceful physical space, we allow ourselves to open the door to a relaxed and peaceful mental space.

All the magic happens in your sacred space, where you enter a state of relaxation and peace. In this state, the clutter of stress and resistance is defeated and released, and the magic tree of ideas starts to take root. When these ideas enter your calm and peaceful mind, you are in a clear enough state to observe, analyze, and take action toward manifesting happiness and creativity in ways beyond your most rampant imaginations.

A sacred space is essential if you wish to optimize your lifestyle. Without a sacred space, Steven King wouldn't have written Carrie to get his start, nor the 100+ books after Carrie. It's worth giving a shot. You'll find a new love you never knew existed.

Here are some ideas for creating your sacred space:

- **Section off an area of your house, yard, garage, closet**, or anywhere else you feel you can achieve the most relaxation and silence. If using an outdoor space, consider a canopy or other type of cover for those beautiful rainy days.
- **Eliminate distractions and clutter** in the space, including excess furniture, televisions, mobile phones (except for music), family, friends, and any other attention-sucking rabbit holes.
- **Hang wall tapestries, artwork, or other high-energy and creative items** which resonate with your energy and motivation.
- **Lay down colorful rugs or yoga blankets, and stack floor pillows** or folded blankets as a sitting platform. Everyone has different preferences, so if you're a floor person, rock that floor! If you're a desk person, rock that desk!
- **Lay other items of meaning and value around** your sacred space to remind you of how awesome life is (pictures, stones, or gems, etc.).
- **Create a vision board and place it where you can see it.** Opening your eyes after a meditation or focus session to all the awesome things you are working toward manifesting in your life will inspire you.

- **Add the three primal elements** to your setting. Introduce a mason jar of water (the elixir of life), air-purifying plants (earth: English Ivy, peace lilies, snake plants, spider plant, aloe, ferns, etc), and some fire (candles, incense, sage, etc).
- **Listen to music that inspires you**. Turn the volume down if in creation or meditation mode.
- **Keep inspirational books or resources that are supportive of your journey** around for digestion, motivation, and deep thinking.
- **Optimize your lighting preference** with bright lights or light dimmers.
- **Decorate your sacred space** with your favorite inspirational quotes, mantras, and memes.
- **Keep writing pads and your journal within reach** to jot down ideas and provide plenty of space for scribbling brain maps, masterminding outlines, and pinpointing your optimized direction!

Add anything else that is meaningful to you and your uniqueness. This space is a place for you to truly disconnect from the distraction-flooded world and connect deeply with your muse, internal hero, and future self!

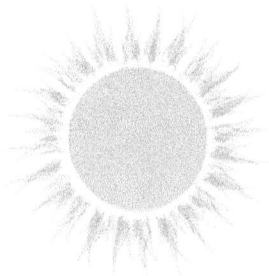

DATE .... / .... / 20 ....

Avoid being boxed in. Go find something
that allows you to breathe.
– Bri Seeley

BG:

Breath of Life

Close your eyes and breathe deeply for as long as possible.

Current Mood: Duration:

Sweet-Ass Affirmations

I am....

What are the two **most valuable actions** I will take today to progress toward my goals, dreams, and optimal health?

1.

2.

What makes me ☺ and why?

Wildcard

Creating a Sacred Space

Set aside a half hour today to plan out or create your sacred space.

Sweet-Ass Reward

How will I reward myself after accomplishing my two valuable actions today?

My **wins** for the day are:

Party Checklist

☐ Rx ☐ Test ☐ Water

☐ Movement ☐ Reward

Breath of Life

Close your eyes and breathe deeply for as long as possible.

Current Mood: Duration:

What are the two **most valuable actions** I will take tomorrow to progress toward my goals, dreams, and optimal health?

1.

2.

Sweet-Ass Affirmations

I am....

Reflection and Thoughts

You are   **12** % done with optimizing your diabetic lifestyle. ☺   **BG:**

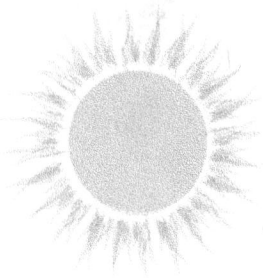

DATE .... / .... / 20 ....

She was afraid of heights, but she was much
more afraid of never flying.
– Atticus

BG:

Breath of Life

Close your eyes and breathe deeply for as long as possible.

Current Mood: Duration:

Sweet-Ass Affirmations

I am....

What are the two **most valuable actions** I will take today to progress toward my goals, dreams, and optimal health?

1.

2.

What makes me ☺ and why?

Wildcard

Knowledge Bomb

Replace your self-criticism with self-compassion.

Sweet-Ass Reward

How will I reward myself after accomplishing my two valuable actions today?

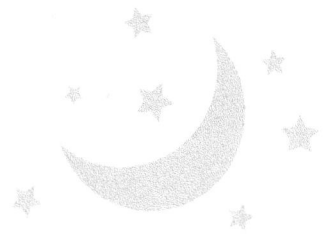

My **wins** for the day are:

Party Checklist

.

☐ Rx ☐ Test ☐ Water

☐ Movement ☐ Reward

Breath of Life

Close your eyes and breathe deeply for as long as possible.

Current Mood: Duration:

What are the two **most valuable actions** I will take tomorrow to progress toward my goals, dreams, and optimal health?

1.

2.

Sweet-Ass Affirmations

I am....

Reflection and Thoughts

You are   **13** % done with optimizing your diabetic lifestyle. ☺   **BG:**

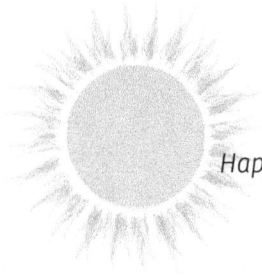

DATE .... / .... / 20 ....

*Happiness is letting go of what you think your life is supposed
to look like and celebrating it for everything that it is.*
– Mandy Hale

BG:

Breath of Life

Close your eyes and breathe deeply for as long as possible.

Current Mood: Duration:

Sweet-Ass Affirmations

I am....

What are the two **most valuable actions** I will take today to progress toward my goals, dreams, and optimal health?

1.

2.

What makes me ☺ and why?

Wildcard

Knowledge Bomb

You are SO MUCH more than a person living with diabetes.

Sweet-Ass Reward

How will I reward myself after accomplishing my two valuable actions today?

My **wins** for the day are:

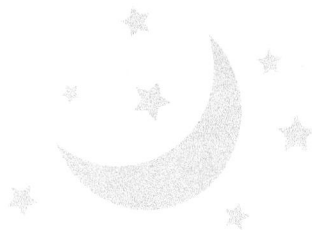

Party Checklist

☐ Rx   ☐ Test   ☐ Water

☐ Movement   ☐ Reward

Breath of Life

Close your eyes and breathe deeply for as long as possible.

Current Mood: Duration:

What are the two **most valuable actions** I will take tomorrow to progress toward my goals, dreams, and optimal health?

1.

2.

Sweet-Ass Affirmations

I am....

Reflection and Thoughts

You are   **14** % done with optimizing your diabetic lifestyle. ☺

BG:

Wildcard: Meal Planning and Nutrition Optimization

Diabetes and nutrition go hand in hand. There is no denying that what we eat, specifically carbohydrates, has a direct correlation with our glucose levels, but that does not mean you have to eat boring and tasteless food! Unfortunately, some people automatically think a "diabetic-friendly" diet is less than desirable and restrictive, when in fact it is eating a healthy variety of food in the appropriate amounts. The "diabetic diet" is one of the healthiest ones out there and should be followed by many!

There are many ways to approach your relationship to food and your diabetes management, one of them being meal planning and preparation. Find one that works for you! By having meals planned and/or prepped ahead of time, you take away the guesswork and the temptation to go for the convenient foods that are less nutrient-dense or healthy.

Since carbohydrates (not sugar, as sugar is a type of carb) are what mainly raises blood glucose levels, another method people find helpful when creating and/or staying on track with their meal plan and nutrition is carb counting. There are many resources in the bonus material to help with carb counting, substitutions, and suggested guidelines, but below are a few quick tips and tricks to get you started with the nutrition that fits you best:

- Opt for baked or steamed lean meats such as fish, chicken, and turkey.
- The more color on your plate, the better.
- Opt for berries if you are reaching for fruit as they are lower in carbs.
- Plan for one meal at a time so you don't become overwhelmed.
- Pair a carb snack or meal with a protein to slow down the absorption of glucose into the bloodstream.
- Schedule meals and snacks around the same times each day to help keep blood sugars level.
- Keep portion sizes in mind.
- Replace late-night snacks with water.
- Do not skip meals.
- Fiber is your friend!

Also, you have a new party favor in the party checklist! When you have created, followed, or maintained your nutrition goals, treat yo' self by checking this box! You can also actually treat yo' self with a delicious meal and snack, too. ☺

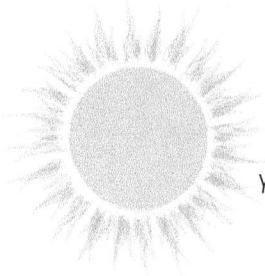

DATE .... / .... / 20 ....

Your day will go the way the corners of your mouth turn.
– Unknown

BG:

Breath of Life

Close your eyes and breathe deeply for as long as possible.

Current Mood: Duration:

Sweet-Ass Affirmations

I am....

What are the two **most valuable actions** I will take today to progress toward my goals, dreams, and optimal health?

1.

2.

What makes me ☺ and why?

Wildcard

Meal Magic

Your body is your sanctuary! Take a few moments today to read through the bonus material on optimal nutrition, meal planning, and recipes. Start your kitchen audit and move forward from there!

Sweet-Ass Reward

How will I reward myself after accomplishing my two valuable actions today?

My **wins** for the day are:

Party Checklist

☐ Rx   ☐ Test   ☐ Water

☐ Nutrition   ☐ Movement   ☐ Reward

Breath of Life

Close your eyes and breathe deeply for as long as possible.

Current Mood: Duration:

What are the two **most valuable actions** I will take tomorrow to progress toward my goals, dreams, and optimal health?

1.

2.

Sweet-Ass Affirmations

I am....

Reflection and Thoughts

You are   **15** % done with optimizing your diabetic lifestyle. ☺   **BG:**

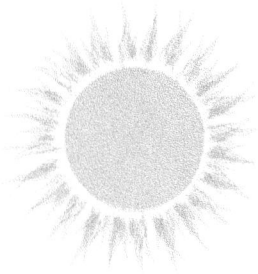

DATE .... / .... / 20 ....

Your worst enemy cannot harm you as much
as your own thoughts, unguarded.
– Buddha

BG:

Breath of Life

Close your eyes and breathe deeply for as long as possible.

Current Mood: Duration:

Sweet-Ass Affirmations

I am....

What are the two **most valuable actions** I will take today to progress toward my goals, dreams, and optimal health?

1.

2.

What makes me ☺ and why?

Wildcard

Knowledge Bomb

Fiber helps manage your blood sugar, keeps you feeling full, and is good for your heart health.

Sweet-Ass Reward

How will I reward myself after accomplishing my two valuable actions today?

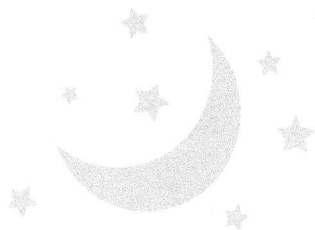

My **wins** for the day are:

Party Checklist

☐ Rx   ☐ Test   ☐ Water
☐ Nutrition   ☐ Movement   ☐ Reward

Breath of Life

Close your eyes and breathe deeply for as long as possible.

Current Mood: Duration:

What are the two **most valuable actions** I will take tomorrow to
progress toward my goals, dreams, and optimal health?

1.

2.

Sweet-Ass Affirmations

I am....

Reflection and Thoughts

BG:

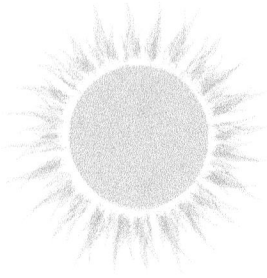

DATE .... / .... / 20 ....

Perfect becomes the enemy of good.
– Orlando Pescetti

BG:

Breath of Life

Close your eyes and breathe deeply for as long as possible.

Current Mood: Duration:

Sweet-Ass Affirmations

I am....

What are the two **most valuable actions** I will take today to progress toward my goals, dreams, and optimal health?

1.

2.

What makes me ☺ and why?

Wildcard

Knowledge Bomb

Try replacing some carbs with good fat such as avocados, nuts, olive oil, and MCT oil.

Sweet-Ass Reward

How will I reward myself after accomplishing my two valuable actions today?

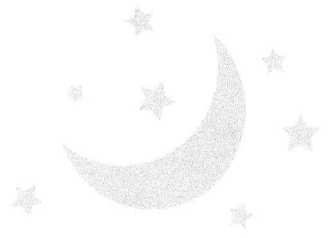

My **wins** for the day are:

Party Checklist

☐ Rx ☐ Test ☐ Water

☐ Nutrition ☐ Movement ☐ Reward

Breath of Life

Close your eyes and breathe deeply for as long as possible.

Current Mood: Duration:

What are the two **most valuable actions** I will take tomorrow to
progress toward my goals, dreams, and optimal health?

1.

2.

Sweet-Ass Affirmations

I am....

Reflection and Thoughts

You are   **17** % done with optimizing your diabetic lifestyle. ☺   **BG:**

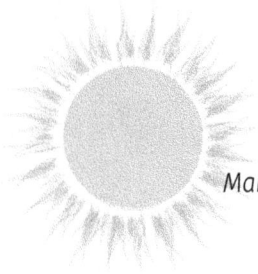

DATE .... / .... / 20 ....

Many wealthy people are merely janitors of their possessions.
– Frank Lloyd Wright

BG:

Breath of Life

Close your eyes and breathe deeply for as long as possible.

Current Mood: Duration:

Sweet-Ass Affirmations

I am....

What are the two **most valuable actions** I will take today to progress toward my goals, dreams, and optimal health?

1.

2.

What makes me ☺ and why?

Wildcard

Knowledge Bomb

Read the portion sizes on nutrition labels.

Sweet-Ass Reward

How will I reward myself after accomplishing my two valuable actions today?

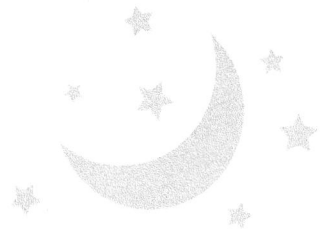

My **wins** for the day are:

Party Checklist

☐ Rx ☐ Test ☐ Water

☐ Nutrition ☐ Movement ☐ Reward

Breath of Life

Close your eyes and breathe deeply for as long as possible.

Current Mood: Duration:

What are the two **most valuable actions** I will take tomorrow to progress toward my goals, dreams, and optimal health?

1.

2.

Sweet-Ass Affirmations

I am....

Reflection and Thoughts

You are **18** % done with optimizing your diabetic lifestyle. ☺   **BG:**

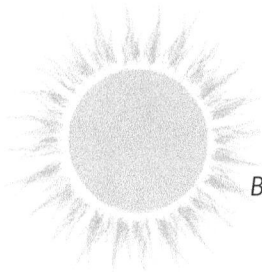

DATE .... / .... / 20 ....

Be somebody that makes everybody feel like a somebody.
– Unknown

BG:

Breath of Life

Close your eyes and breathe deeply for as long as possible.

Current Mood: Duration:

Sweet-Ass Affirmations

I am....

What are the two **most valuable actions** I will take today to progress toward my goals, dreams, and optimal health?

1.

2.

What makes me ☺ and why?

Wildcard

Exercise / Movement

Have you moved that sexy body yet today? Choose a few exercises on your own or from the bonus material and get that blood flowing!

Sweet-Ass Reward

How will I reward myself after accomplishing my two valuable actions today?

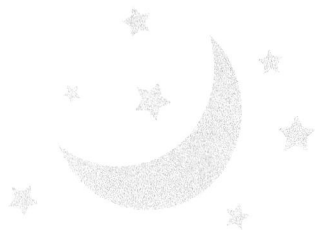

My **wins** for the day are:

Party Checklist

☐ Rx   ☐ Test   ☐ Water
☐ Nutrition   ☐ Movement   ☐ Reward

Breath of Life

Close your eyes and breathe deeply for as long as possible.

Current Mood: Duration:

What are the two **most valuable actions** I will take tomorrow to
progress toward my goals, dreams, and optimal health?

1.

2.

Sweet-Ass Affirmations

I am....

Reflection and Thoughts

You are **19**% done with optimizing your diabetic lifestyle. ☺

BG:

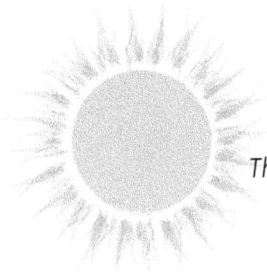

DATE .... / .... / 20 ....

The problem is people are being hated when they are real,
and are being loved when they are fake.
– Bob Marley

BG:

Breath of Life

Close your eyes and breathe deeply for as long as possible.

Current Mood: Duration:

Sweet-Ass Affirmations

I am....

What are the two **most valuable actions** I will take today to progress toward my goals, dreams, and optimal health?

1.

2.

What makes me ☺ and why?

Wildcard

Knowledge Bomb

If plain water isn't your jam, try a fizzy, flavored (but not sweetened) water.

Sweet-Ass Reward

How will I reward myself after accomplishing my two valuable actions today?

My **wins** for the day are:

Party Checklist

☐ Rx   ☐ Test   ☐ Water

☐ Nutrition   ☐ Movement   ☐ Reward

Breath of Life

Close your eyes and breathe deeply for as long as possible.

Current Mood: Duration:

What are the two **most valuable actions** I will take tomorrow to progress toward my goals, dreams, and optimal health?

1.

2.

Sweet-Ass Affirmations

I am....

Reflection and Thoughts

You are   20 % done with optimizing your diabetic lifestyle. ☺

BG:

Wildcard: 7-Day Giving Challenge

As media and marketing flood our brains with the idea that success is defined by how much we earn, many of us rate our happiness based on the materialistic belongings and monetary value we stack up. As soon as we receive something, we immediately start craving even more! We are rarely content with what we already have. Having a desire for more is a great characteristic when it comes to creativity and developing the self, but a terrible characteristic when it comes to stacking our cheese and junk piles.

We are not arguing that receiving gifts, raises, and nicer things doesn't make us feel good momentarily, but it doesn't create and sustain happiness long-term. If receiving more of everything isn't the answer to happiness, then what is?

Giving!

When you give something to another person, whether material or in service, a physiological response happens within you. That warm, fuzzy feeling comes back, and it lets you make sexy time with your happiness muscle. Your brain releases pleasure endorphins, including oxytocin, which is also released during sex and lowers your stress. Oxytocin also makes you feel more connected to others, which is why people often pay forward random acts of kindness. We bet there has been a time in your life when someone did something nice for you or even gave you a gift without an occasion. In return, you paid it forward to someone else when you had the chance! It's a domino cycle of warm, fuzzy feelings that increases the bond of the world!

For seven days in a row, and then sporadically over the next 100 days, we challenge you to give a gift, good deed, or other thoughtful exchange to family members, friends, strangers, or even the world as a whole without expecting anything in return. In our experience, this is the #1 practice to sustain happiness, not only in the moment, but long term.

Here are some ideas for giving gifts and good deeds:

- When you reach your minimalist challenge later in this journal, see if any of the items are of value to anyone you know.
- Invite the neighbors over for a casual meal.
- Buy a coffee for the person behind you at a coffee shop.
- Write a thank-you note to someone who has been influential or important in your life.

- Call your family and friends and tell them you love them.
- Volunteer at the local retirement homes and homeless shelters.
- Pick up trash on the side of the road if you stumble upon it.
- Offer your seat to someone else on the crowded bus or subway.
- Help someone who is less fortunate or in need of food, clothing, or shelter.
- Make contributions to charities of your choice (doing this anonymously is even better!). We suggest The Ryan Banks Academy (**www.ryanbanksacademy. org**) if you need a trustworthy, magical place to donate to.
- Buy someone a gym membership.
- Take a piece of dessert to someone at work.
- Give someone a free corndog (advice from Kid President).
- Pick some fresh flowers for your significant other (dudes like flowers, too!).
- Send an email to an old teacher or friend.
- Plant some trees.
- Mow your neighbor's lawn.
- Forgive someone you may be holding a grudge against.
- Offer to babysit for someone, so they can go out and enjoy themselves for a night.
- Give someone an album that you enjoy.
- Take someone on vacation with you (if you have travel points, you could use those!).
- If you have a garden, share the fruits and vegetables with others.
- Give a copy of this journal to someone else!

As you experience this process, we encourage you to keep the habit rolling far beyond the 7-day streak. You will see what kind of magic the world returns to you just for putting your magic into the world. It is also a fantastic process to journal about the gifts and the experience, and there is space in the wildcard box to do this if you wish. Infinite warm, fuzzy feelings await you!

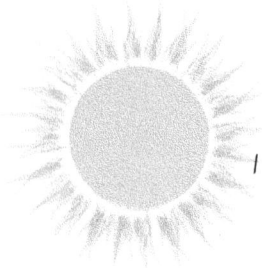

DATE .... / .... / 20 ....

I am an old man who has known a great deal of troubles,
most of which never happened.
– Mark Twain

BG:

Breath of Life

Close your eyes and breathe deeply for as long as possible.

Current Mood: Duration:

Sweet-Ass Affirmations

I am....

What are the two **most valuable actions** I will take today to progress toward my goals, dreams, and optimal health?

1.

2.

What makes me ☺ and why?

Wildcard

Giving Challenge Day 1

What will I give today to impact someone's life in a positive way?

Sweet-Ass Reward

How will I reward myself after accomplishing my two valuable actions today?

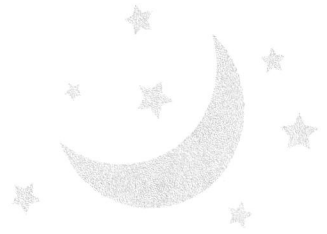

My **wins** for the day are:

Party Checklist

☐ Rx   ☐ Test   ☐ Water
☐ Nutrition   ☐ Movement   ☐ Reward

Breath of Life

Close your eyes and breathe deeply for as long as possible.

Current Mood: Duration:

What are the two **most valuable actions** I will take tomorrow to progress toward my goals, dreams, and optimal health?

1.

2.

Sweet-Ass Affirmations

I am....

Reflection and Thoughts

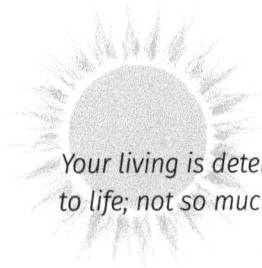

DATE .... / .... / 20 ....

Your living is determined not so much by what life brings to you as by the attitude you bring to life; not so much by what happens to you as by the way your mind looks at what happens.
– Kahlil Gibran

BG:

Breath of Life

Close your eyes and breathe deeply for as long as possible.

Current Mood: Duration:

Sweet-Ass Affirmations

I am....

What are the two **most valuable actions** I will take today to progress toward my goals, dreams, and optimal health?

1.

2.

What makes me ☺ and why?

Wildcard

Giving Challenge Day 2

What will I give today to impact someone's life in a positive way?

Sweet-Ass Reward

How will I reward myself after accomplishing my two valuable actions today?

My **wins** for the day are:

Party Checklist

☐ Rx   ☐ Test   ☐ Water

☐ Nutrition   ☐ Movement   ☐ Reward

Breath of Life

Close your eyes and breathe deeply for as long as possible.

Current Mood: Duration:

What are the two **most valuable actions** I will take tomorrow to progress toward my goals, dreams, and optimal health?

1.

2.

Sweet-Ass Affirmations

I am....

Reflection and Thoughts

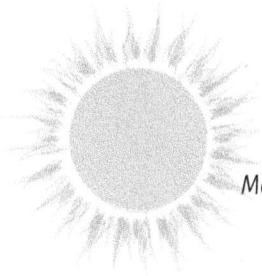

DATE .... / .... / 20 ....

Most folks are as happy as they make up their minds to be.
– Abraham Lincoln

BG:

Breath of Life

Close your eyes and breathe deeply for as long as possible.

Current Mood: Duration:

Sweet-Ass Affirmations

I am....

What are the two **most valuable actions** I will take today to progress toward my goals, dreams, and optimal health?

1.

2.

What makes me ☺ and why?

Wildcard

Giving Challenge Day 3

What will I give today to impact someone's life in a positive way?

Sweet-Ass Reward

How will I reward myself after accomplishing my two valuable actions today?

My **wins** for the day are:

Party Checklist

☐ Rx   ☐ Test   ☐ Water

☐ Nutrition   ☐ Movement   ☐ Reward

Breath of Life

Close your eyes and breathe deeply for as long as possible.

Current Mood: Duration:

What are the two **most valuable actions** I will take tomorrow to progress toward my goals, dreams, and optimal health?

1.

2.

Sweet-Ass Affirmations

I am....

Reflection and Thoughts

You are   23 % done with optimizing your diabetic lifestyle. ☺   **BG:**

DATE .... / .... / 20 ....

Kites rise highest against the wind, not with it.
– Winston Churchill

BG:

Breath of Life

Close your eyes and breathe deeply for as long as possible.

Current Mood: Duration:

Sweet-Ass Affirmations

I am....

What are the two **most valuable actions** I will take today to progress toward my goals, dreams, and optimal health?

1.

2.

What makes me ☺ and why?

Wildcard

Giving Challenge Day 4

What will I give today to impact someone's life in a positive way?

Sweet-Ass Reward

How will I reward myself after accomplishing my two valuable actions today?

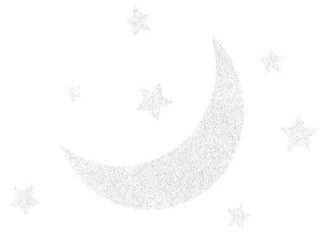

My **wins** for the day are:

Party Checklist

☐ Rx ☐ Test ☐ Water

☐ Nutrition ☐ Movement ☐ Reward

Breath of Life

Close your eyes and breathe deeply for as long as possible.

Current Mood: Duration:

What are the two **most valuable actions** I will take tomorrow to progress toward my goals, dreams, and optimal health?

1.

2.

Sweet-Ass Affirmations

I am....

Reflection and Thoughts

You are **24** % done with optimizing your diabetic lifestyle. ☺

BG:

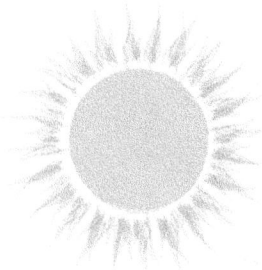

DATE .... / .... / 20 ....

*How wonderful it is that nobody need wait a single
moment before beginning to improve the world.*
– Anne Frank

BG:

Breath of Life

Close your eyes and breathe deeply for as long as possible.

Current Mood: Duration:

Sweet-Ass Affirmations

I am....

What are the two **most valuable actions**
I will take today to progress toward my
goals, dreams, and optimal health?

1.

2.

What makes me ☺ and why?

Wildcard

Giving Challenge Day 5

What will I give today to impact
someone's life in a positive way?

Sweet-Ass Reward

How will I reward myself after accomplishing
my two valuable actions today?

116

My **wins** for the day are:

Party Checklist

☐ Rx   ☐ Test   ☐ Water

☐ Nutrition   ☐ Movement   ☐ Reward

Breath of Life

Close your eyes and breathe deeply for as long as possible.

Current Mood: Duration:

What are the two **most valuable actions** I will take tomorrow to progress toward my goals, dreams, and optimal health?

1.

2.

Sweet-Ass Affirmations

I am....

Reflection and Thoughts

You are   25 % done with optimizing your diabetic lifestyle. ☺   **BG:**

Sweet-Ass 100-Day Visions: Quarterly Review

Wahoo! You champion! You have made it through the first 25 days of journaling, which means you are 25% done with developing your optimal happiness and diabetic lifestyle.

Throughout the 100-day process, we have created quarterly reviews to give you a chance to review the visions you set at the beginning of the journaling process.

Do your visions still feel relevant to the direction you wish to go? How much progress have you made toward your visions? Have you been completing your daily actions to support and achieve your visions? Who knows, maybe you've already manifested one into existence! :)

You may want to revise, replace, or improve parts of your original vision list. That's totally okay! If not, that's also amazing! Every day you are raging closer and closer to bringing your vision to reality.

Below, take a moment to write out your three updated visions. Remember to write them in the present or past tense, as if you are achieving or have already achieved them!

My sweet-ass visions are:

- ....
- ....
- ....

As you sow, so shall you reap. Everything you desire is on its way to you at warp speed!

Join our Patreon Community!

Eazy. Breezy. Diabeezy!

Since you made it this far, we know you are serious about optimizing your diabetic health and expanding your feel-good lifestyle. We are happy to have been able to support you with this journal.

As we grow the Party Like A Diabetic community, we are also eternally grateful for your support and interaction. Just by purchasing this journal, you have helped expand our resources to reach new diabetics in need.

We have created an exclusive Patreon community and want to invite you to join and help grow this mission!

As a Patreon supporter, you will get access to the following:

- **Premium health tips, articles, and tools** about various topics for personal optimization
- **Live group/mastermind video calls** to engage with us and other members, including ongoing interviews with other authors, entrepreneurs, and medical experts
- **Community forum** where you can engage with other Diabadasses.
- **Exclusive bonus content**, including topics revolving around nutrition, diet planning, habit creation, happiness, exercise and more.
- **Discounts and early access** to new products (help us with beta testing!)
- **Meetups, parties, and local events** for our community!
- **Unlimited smiles**

We can't wait to party with you!

Join today: **www.sweetassjournal.com/pladpatreon**

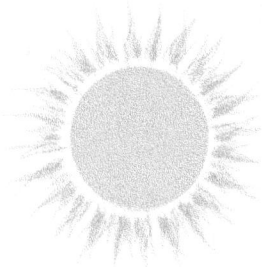

DATE .... / .... / 20 ....

The gem cannot be polished without friction,
nor man perfected without trials.
– Confucius

BG:

Breath of Life

Close your eyes and breathe deeply for as long as possible.

Current Mood: Duration:

Sweet-Ass Affirmations

I am....

What are the two **most valuable actions** I will take today to progress toward my goals, dreams, and optimal health?

1.

2.

What makes me ☺ and why?

Wildcard

Giving Challenge Day 6

What will I give today to impact someone's life in a positive way?

Sweet-Ass Reward

How will I reward myself after accomplishing my two valuable actions today?

My **wins** for the day are:

Party Checklist

☐ Rx   ☐ Test   ☐ Water

☐ Nutrition   ☐ Movement   ☐ Reward

Breath of Life

Close your eyes and breathe deeply for as long as possible.

Current Mood: Duration:

What are the two **most valuable actions** I will take tomorrow to
progress toward my goals, dreams, and optimal health?

1.

2.

Sweet-Ass Affirmations

I am....

Reflection and Thoughts

You are **26** % done with optimizing your diabetic lifestyle. ☺   **BG:**

DATE .... / .... / 20 ....

A pessimist sees the difficulty in every opportunity;
an optimist sees the opportunity in every difficulty.
– Winston Churchill

BG:

Breath of Life

Close your eyes and breathe deeply for as long as possible.

Current Mood: Duration:

Sweet-Ass Affirmations

I am....

What are the two **most valuable actions** I will take today to progress toward my goals, dreams, and optimal health?

1.

2.

What makes me ☺ and why?

Wildcard

Giving Challenge Day 7

What will I give today to impact someone's life in a positive way?

Sweet-Ass Reward

How will I reward myself after accomplishing my two valuable actions today?

My **wins** for the day are:

Party Checklist

☐ Rx   ☐ Test   ☐ Water

☐ Nutrition   ☐ Movement   ☐ Reward

Breath of Life

Close your eyes and breathe deeply for as long as possible.

Current Mood: Duration:

What are the two **most valuable actions** I will take tomorrow to progress toward my goals, dreams, and optimal health?

1.

2.

Sweet-Ass Affirmations

I am....

Reflection and Thoughts

BG:

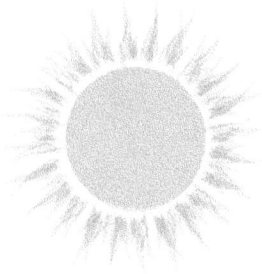

DATE .... / .... / 20 ....

You have to assemble life yourself, action by action.
– Marcus Aurelius

BG:

Breath of Life

Close your eyes and breathe deeply for as long as possible.

Current Mood: Duration:

Sweet-Ass Affirmations

I am....

What are the two **most valuable actions** I will take today to progress toward my goals, dreams, and optimal health?

1.

2.

What makes me ☺ and why?

Wildcard

Knowledge Bomb

Staying connected with the diabetic community is a great way to stay positive, learn, and feel understood.

Join our diabetic facebook community by accessing your free bonus materials at:
www.sweetassjournal.com/pladbonus

Sweet-Ass Reward

How will I reward myself after accomplishing my two valuable actions today?

My **wins** for the day are:

Party Checklist

☐ Rx ☐ Test ☐ Water

☐ Nutrition ☐ Movement ☐ Reward

Breath of Life

Close your eyes and breathe deeply for as long as possible.

Current Mood: Duration:

What are the two **most valuable actions** I will take tomorrow to progress toward my goals, dreams, and optimal health?

1.

2.

Sweet-Ass Affirmations

I am....

Reflection and Thoughts

You are 28 % done with optimizing your diabetic lifestyle. ☺   **BG:**

Wildcard: Abundance Lists—I have an abundance of...

Just as we celebrate our wins to reflect on our momentum and juice up our motivation, it is equally important to celebrate our abundance.

We have already stressed the importance of practicing gratitude for all that you have. It is also important to express gratitude for the valuable mental and physical allies you have fighting next to you, sustaining and supporting you while you work toward more meaningful and powerful experiences. The people around you who support your journey are vital contributors to your mission!

People think of money most often when they hear the term **abundance**. Although money is an incredible form of abundance, people, materials, skillsets, experiences, and even the basic elements of life—everything supporting your journey—are also your abundance. You must pause and reflect often on just how big and beautiful your arsenal of abundance is so you can defeat the poisonous mindset gremlins when they try to convince you that you don't have enough.

These gremlins often whisper atrocious things into your thoughts, like, "If I just had a little more time, I could do these awesome things." Or, "If I just had a little more money, I could afford to do these awesome things." Or, "If I just had someone to help me, I'd be able to do these awesome things." They want you to focus on what you don't have. They want you to feel like you are limited in your abilities. They throw New Year-caliber parties with oodles of disco balls every time you fail to be grateful for what you already have.

Remember, focusing on the negative will only breed more negativity into your life. Following the anti-abundance gremlins will lead you down a dead-end alley where you will get mugged by limitation.

You *must* understand that you have anything and everything you need, right now, to develop into a happier, more valuable, sweet-ass version of you!

From now on, the wildcard box may present you with an "I have an abundance of..." space. In this section, write down anything and everything in your life that supports you in your journey. These are the seeds of your abundance, and they will only sprout and grow into trees without limitation if you recognize their existence and support them! You can even take it a step further and write out how the abundance of 'X' impacts your life. There is no wrong way to do this, so be as simple or detailed as you wish!

Some examples to get your abundance mind flowing:

I have an abundance of...

- energy which allows me to create
- sunlight which allows me to re-energize
- fresh air which allows me to breathe
- family members who support me
- transportation available to me
- free resources online to help me learn anything imaginable
- time to relax and enjoy the company of my loved ones
- water available to me for drinking, hygiene, and washing my abundance of clothes
- undies
- support on my diabetic journey
- money because I am alive and able to care for myself
- honey and tea to help kickstart the day
- Arnold Schwarzenegger merchandise
- trails, mountains, lakes, trees, and parks around me where I can bond with the great outdoors
- skills which allow me to support myself and my family
- awesome people who will soon come into my life
- gifts I can give others to brighten up their day
- outlets to charge my electronics
- resting places to rejuvenate the mind and body
- dreams which I am manifesting
- happiness and creativity
- opportunity ahead of me

As you practice your abundance list, you will quickly shape your awareness around all the positive support in your life. Always shift your focus from what you don't have to what you do have. When you think positively, you will breed more positivity. Make sexy-time with your abundance and pop out some positive juju babies. You are in a position to be as happy and free as you decide to be, and your abundance will grow alongside you.

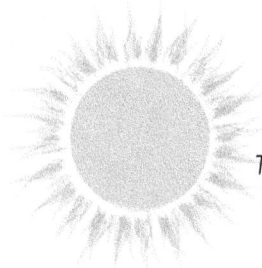

DATE .... / .... / 20 ....

The best teachers are those who show you where to look,
but don't tell you what to see.
– Alexandra K. Trenfor

BG:

Breath of Life

Close your eyes and breathe deeply for as long as possible.

Current Mood: Duration:

Sweet-Ass Affirmations

· I am....

What are the two **most valuable actions** I will take today to progress toward my goals, dreams, and optimal health?

1.

2.

What makes me ☺ and why?

Wildcard

Abundance List

I have an abundance of:

Sweet-Ass Reward

How will I reward myself after accomplishing my two valuable actions today?

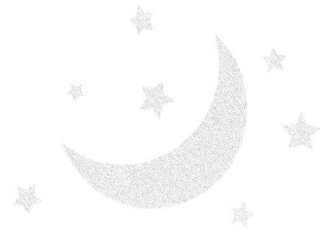

My **wins** for the day are:

Party Checklist

☐ Rx ☐ Test ☐ Water

☐ Nutrition ☐ Movement ☐ Reward

Breath of Life

Close your eyes and breathe deeply for as long as possible.

Current Mood: Duration:

What are the two **most valuable actions** I will take tomorrow to progress toward my goals, dreams, and optimal health?

1.

2.

Sweet-Ass Affirmations

I am....

Reflection and Thoughts

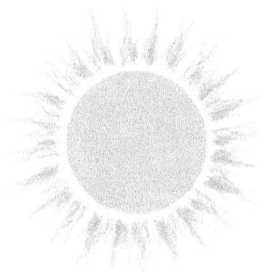

DATE .... / .... / 20 ....

Be happy in the moment, that's enough.
Each moment is all we need, not more.
– Mother Teresa

BG:

Breath of Life

Close your eyes and breathe deeply for as long as possible.

Current Mood: Duration:

Sweet-Ass Affirmations

I am....

What are the two **most valuable actions** I will take today to progress toward my goals, dreams, and optimal health?

1.

2.

What makes me ☺ and why?

Wildcard

Knowledge Bomb

Thoughts, feelings, beliefs, and attitudes affect how healthy your body is.

Sweet-Ass Reward

How will I reward myself after accomplishing my two valuable actions today?

130

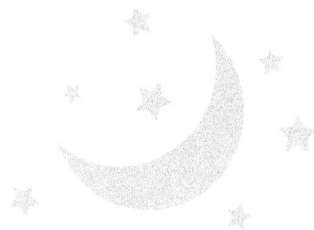

My **wins** for the day are:

Party Checklist

☐ Rx ☐ Test ☐ Water

☐ Nutrition ☐ Movement ☐ Reward

Breath of Life

Close your eyes and breathe deeply for as long as possible.

Current Mood: Duration:

What are the two **most valuable actions** I will take tomorrow to progress toward my goals, dreams, and optimal health?

1.

2.

Sweet-Ass Affirmations

I am....

Reflection and Thoughts

You are **30** % done with optimizing your diabetic lifestyle. ☺

BG:

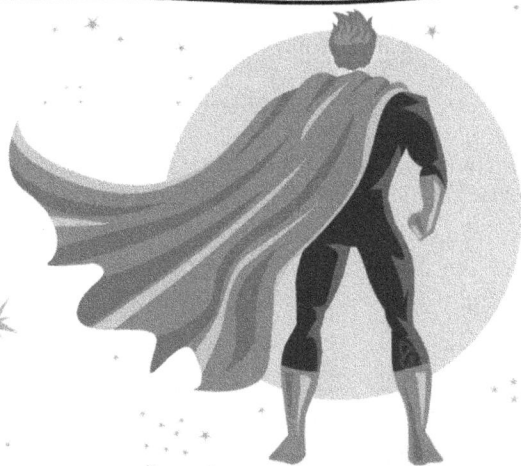

I AM THE HERO IN MY OWN VIDEO GAME.

You are leveling up. You are gaining superpowers. You bust through brick walls and smash the skulls of fear gremlins around every corner. You fall off cliffs. You get attacked and eaten by monsters. But, you always show back up twice as strong, mentored by the wisdom of your wounds. Bust through the levels! Throw fireballs at all that resists, and blindside the boss who holds your passion hostage! Free the royalty within and conquer your creative empire. Be the last action hero.

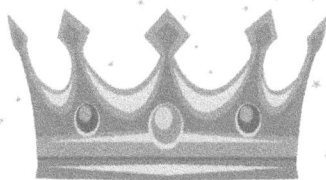

Rage Create

DATE .... / .... / 20 ....

You owe yourself the love that you so
freely give to other people.
– Alexandra Elle

BG:

Breath of Life

Close your eyes and breathe deeply for as long as possible.

Current Mood: Duration:

Sweet-Ass Affirmations

I am....

What are the two **most valuable actions** I will take today to progress toward my goals, dreams, and optimal health?

1.

2.

What makes me ☺ and why?

Wildcard

Meal Magic

Your body is your sanctuary! Write down everything you consume throughout your day to analyze how your nutritional intake affects your blood sugar readings.

Sweet-Ass Reward

How will I reward myself after accomplishing my two valuable actions today?

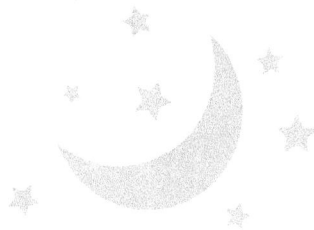

My **wins** for the day are:

Party Checklist

☐ Rx ☐ Test ☐ Water

☐ Nutrition ☐ Movement ☐ Reward

Breath of Life

Close your eyes and breathe deeply for as long as possible.

Current Mood: Duration:

What are the two **most valuable actions** I will take tomorrow to
progress toward my goals, dreams, and optimal health?

1.

2.

Sweet-Ass Affirmations

I am....

Reflection and Thoughts

You are   **31** % done with optimizing your diabetic lifestyle. ☺

BG:

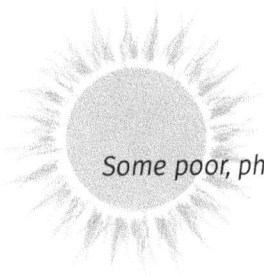

DATE .... / .... / 20 ....

Some poor, phoneless fool is probably sitting next to a waterfall somewhere totally unaware of how angry and scared he's suppose to be.
– Duncan Trussell

BG:

Breath of Life

Close your eyes and breathe deeply for as long as possible.

Current Mood: Duration:

Sweet-Ass Affirmations

I am....

What are the two **most valuable actions** I will take today to progress toward my goals, dreams, and optimal health?

1.

2.

What makes me ☺ and why?

Wildcard

Knowledge Bomb

Stay hydrated! Dehydration can cause higher blood glucose levels.

Sweet-Ass Reward

How will I reward myself after accomplishing my two valuable actions today?

My **wins** for the day are:

Party Checklist

☐ Rx   ☐ Test   ☐ Water

☐ Nutrition   ☐ Movement   ☐ Reward

Breath of Life

Close your eyes and breathe deeply for as long as possible.

Current Mood: Duration:

What are the two **most valuable actions** I will take tomorrow to progress toward my goals, dreams, and optimal health?

1.

2.

Sweet-Ass Affirmations

I am....

Reflection and Thoughts

You are   **32** % done with optimizing your diabetic lifestyle. ☺

BG:

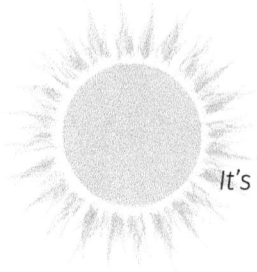

DATE .... / .... / 20 ....

It's easy to be miserable. Being happy is tougher— and cooler.
– Thom Yorke

BG:

Breath of Life

Close your eyes and breathe deeply for as long as possible.

Current Mood: Duration:

Sweet-Ass Affirmations

I am....

What are the two **most valuable actions** I will take today to progress toward my goals, dreams, and optimal health?

1.

2.

What makes me ☺ and why?

Wildcard

Knowledge Bomb

Keep fast-acting carbs nearby during exercise or movement to prevent low blood sugar episodes.

Sweet-Ass Reward

How will I reward myself after accomplishing my two valuable actions today?

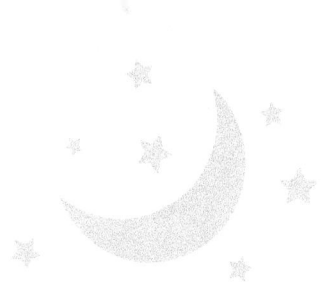

My **wins** for the day are:

Party Checklist

☐ Rx   ☐ Test   ☐ Water

☐ Nutrition   ☐ Movement   ☐ Reward

Breath of Life

Close your eyes and breathe deeply for as long as possible.

Current Mood: Duration:

What are the two **most valuable actions** I will take tomorrow to progress toward my goals, dreams, and optimal health?

1.

2.

Sweet-Ass Affirmations

I am....

Reflection and Thoughts

You are   **33** % done with optimizing your diabetic lifestyle. ☺

BG:

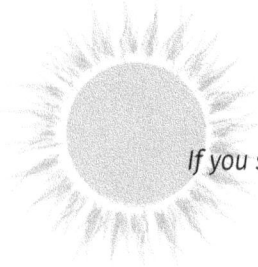

DATE .... / .... / 20 ....

If you stay loyal to your passion, you will live the life of your dreams.
If you don't, there's no way you can.
– Dave Lent

BG:

Breath of Life

Close your eyes and breathe deeply for as long as possible.

Current Mood: Duration:

Sweet-Ass Affirmations

I am....

What are the two **most valuable actions** I will take today to progress toward my goals, dreams, and optimal health?

1.

2.

What makes me ☺ and why?

Wildcard

Knowledge Bomb

Find a friend to work out with for both accountability and fun.

Sweet-Ass Reward

How will I reward myself after accomplishing my two valuable actions today?

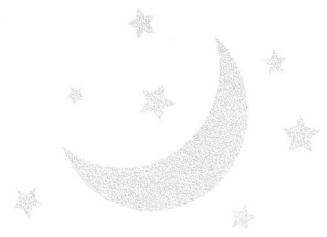

My **wins** for the day are:

Breath of Life

Close your eyes and breathe deeply for as long as possible.

Current Mood: Duration:

What are the two **most valuable actions** I will take tomorrow to progress toward my goals, dreams, and optimal health?

1.

2.

Sweet-Ass Affirmations

I am....

Reflection and Thoughts

You are   **34** % done with optimizing your diabetic lifestyle. ☺

BG:

Wildcard: Brainstorming Ideas

Starting today, and sporadically throughout the rest of the journal, we have included prompts in the wildcard box for you to generate ideas based on specific topics. These boxes are pretty straightforward: list as many ideas as you can that flood into your brain. The quality of your ideas does not matter. It's about being persistent in generating them. There will be a mass of ideas that are bogus material, but there will also be sunshine and star material! If you keep showing up, you'll eventually birth a golden nugget!

Writing down ideas consistently helps build your idea muscle. As this muscle gets stronger, you will become more creative and efficient in brainstorming and problem solving. Some of these ideas will become a special part of your journey to awaken your happiness and optimize your life.

In a way, ideas are sent to you from your muse! They are dreams that want to be manifested. They are projects that want to be physically birthed onto the earth! If you make a partnership with the right ideas, you will continue to accelerate toward your optimal self.

Go ahead! Get started!

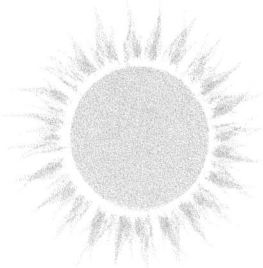

DATE .... / .... / 20 ....

The question isn't 'Who's going to let me?' it's,
'Who's going to stop me?'
– Ayn Rand

BG:

Breath of Life

Close your eyes and breathe deeply for as long as possible.

Current Mood: Duration:

Sweet-Ass Affirmations

I am....

What are the two **most valuable actions** I will take today to progress toward my goals, dreams, and optimal health?

1.

2.

What makes me ☺ and why?

Wildcard

Idea Muscle

Brainstorm a few ideas for overcoming diabetes burnout:

View suggestions in the bonus material at:
www.sweetassjournal.com/pladbonus

Sweet-Ass Reward

How will I reward myself after accomplishing my two valuable actions today?

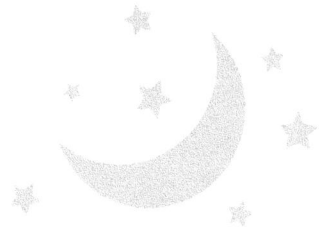

My **wins** for the day are:

Party Checklist

☐ Rx   ☐ Test   ☐ Water

☐ Nutrition   ☐ Movement   ☐ Reward

Breath of Life

Close your eyes and breathe deeply for as long as possible.

Current Mood: Duration:

What are the two **most valuable actions** I will take tomorrow to progress toward my goals, dreams, and optimal health?

1.

2.

Sweet-Ass Affirmations

I am....

Reflection and Thoughts

You are   35 % done with optimizing your diabetic lifestyle. ☺

BG:

DATE .... / .... / 20 ....

Holding onto resentment is like holding your breath.
Only you suffocate.
– Deepak Chopra

BG:

Breath of Life

Close your eyes and breathe deeply for as long as possible.

Current Mood: Duration:

Sweet-Ass Affirmations

I am....

What are the two **most valuable actions** I will take today to progress toward my goals, dreams, and optimal health?

1.

2.

What makes me ☺ and why?

Wildcard

Knowledge Bomb

Instead of packing a cooler with traditional ice packs, pick a cool pack (ex: Frio) that doesn't require freezing or refrigeration.

Sweet-Ass Reward

How will I reward myself after accomplishing my two valuable actions today?

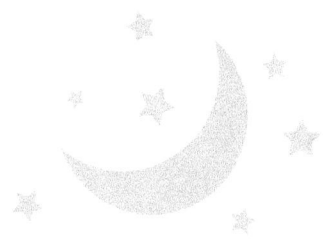

My **wins** for the day are:

Party Checklist

☐ Rx   ☐ Test   ☐ Water

☐ Nutrition   ☐ Movement   ☐ Reward

Breath of Life

Close your eyes and breathe deeply for as long as possible.

Current Mood: Duration:

What are the two **most valuable actions** I will take tomorrow to
progress toward my goals, dreams, and optimal health?

1.

2.

Sweet-Ass Affirmations

I am....

Reflection and Thoughts

You are   **36** % done with optimizing your diabetic lifestyle. ☺

BG:

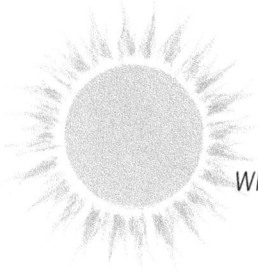

DATE ………… / ………… / 20 …………

Whether you think you can, or think you can't - you're right.
– Henry Ford

BG:

Breath of Life

Close your eyes and breathe deeply for as long as possible.

Current Mood: Duration:

Sweet-Ass Affirmations

I am....

What are the two **most valuable actions** I will take today to progress toward my goals, dreams, and optimal health?

1.

2.

What makes me ☺ and why?

Wildcard

Abundance List

I have an abundance of:

Sweet-Ass Reward

How will I reward myself after accomplishing my two valuable actions today?

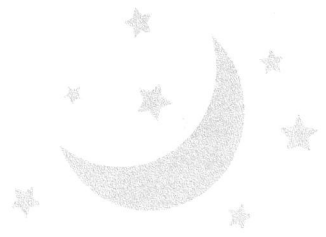

My **wins** for the day are:

Breath of Life

Close your eyes and breathe deeply for as long as possible.

Current Mood: Duration:

What are the two **most valuable actions** I will take tomorrow to progress toward my goals, dreams, and optimal health?

1.

2.

Sweet-Ass Affirmations

I am....

Reflection and Thoughts

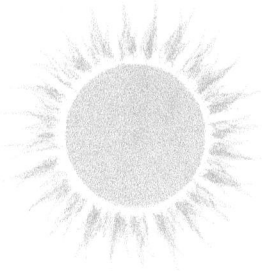

DATE .... / .... / 20 ....

Things turn out the best for those that make
the best of the way things turn out.
– John Wooden

BG:

Breath of Life

Close your eyes and breathe deeply for as long as possible.

Current Mood: Duration:

Sweet-Ass Affirmations

I am....

What are the two **most valuable actions** I will take today to progress toward my goals, dreams, and optimal health?

1.

2.

What makes me ☺ and why?

Wildcard

Knowledge Bomb

Pack a carry-on while flying so your supplies are always with you.

Sweet-Ass Reward

How will I reward myself after accomplishing my two valuable actions today?

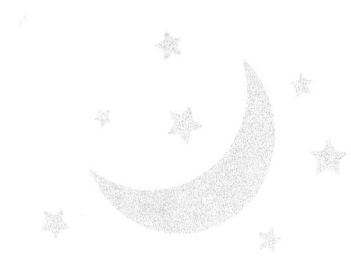

My **wins** for the day are:

Party Checklist

☐ Rx   ☐ Test   ☐ Water

☐ Nutrition   ☐ Movement   ☐ Reward

Breath of Life

Close your eyes and breathe deeply for as long as possible.

Current Mood: Duration:

What are the two **most valuable actions** I will take tomorrow to progress toward my goals, dreams, and optimal health?

1.

2.

Sweet-Ass Affirmations

I am....

Reflection and Thoughts

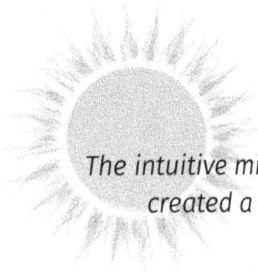

DATE .... / .... / 20 ....

The intuitive mind is a sacred gift, and the rational mind is a faithful servant. We have created a society that honors the servant and has forgotten the sacred gift.
– Albert Einstein

BG:

Breath of Life

Close your eyes and breathe deeply for as long as possible.

Current Mood: Duration:

Sweet-Ass Affirmations

I am....

What are the two **most valuable actions** I will take today to progress toward my goals, dreams, and optimal health?

1.

2.

What makes me ☺ and why?

Wildcard

Giving Challenge

What will I give today to impact someone's life in a positive way?

Sweet-Ass Reward

How will I reward myself after accomplishing my two valuable actions today?

My **wins** for the day are:

Party Checklist

☐ Rx   ☐ Test   ☐ Water

☐ Nutrition   ☐ Movement   ☐ Reward

Breath of Life

Close your eyes and breathe deeply for as long as possible.

Current Mood: Duration:

What are the two **most valuable actions** I will take tomorrow to
progress toward my goals, dreams, and optimal health?

1.

2.

Sweet-Ass Affirmations

I am....

Reflection and Thoughts

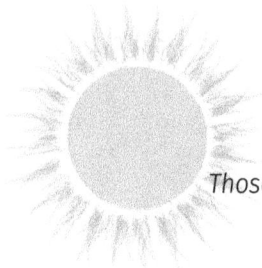

DATE .... / .... / 20 ....

Those people who tried to bury you didn't know you were a seed.
– Unknown

BG:

Breath of Life

Close your eyes and breathe deeply for as long as possible.

Current Mood: Duration:

Sweet-Ass Affirmations

I am....

What are the two **most valuable actions** I will take today to progress toward my goals, dreams, and optimal health?

1.

2.

What makes me ☺ and why?

Wildcard

Exercise / Movement

Have you moved that sexy body yet today? Choose a few exercises on your own or from the bonus material and get that blood flowing!

Sweet-Ass Reward

How will I reward myself after accomplishing my two valuable actions today?

My **wins** for the day are:

Party Checklist

☐ Rx   ☐ Test   ☐ Water

☐ Nutrition   ☐ Movement   ☐ Reward

Breath of Life

Close your eyes and breathe deeply for as long as possible.

Current Mood: Duration:

What are the two **most valuable actions** I will take tomorrow to progress toward my goals, dreams, and optimal health?

1.

2.

Sweet-Ass Affirmations

I am....

Reflection and Thoughts

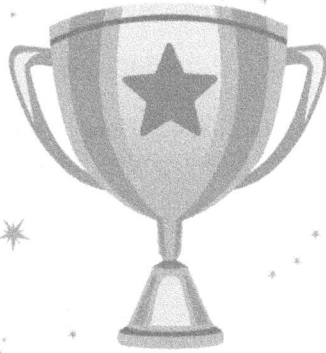

I LIVE EACH MOMENT
WITH SHINING INTENT.
I AM A
CHAMPION
OF THE SUN.

Do not make the mistake of simply existing as a hermit on the shore, sipping margaritas and never leaving the security of your shell. Kick it into beast mode and dive into the waters. You are the King of Tides. You are the Queen of Light.
You are a maniac banshee doing backflips through the treetops of resistance.
You are a battleship smashing through waves, exploring new lands, and digging up treasures buried deep beneath the comfort beaches. You have breakdowns. You have scars. But you also have wisdom of gold. You are truly alive and full of light.

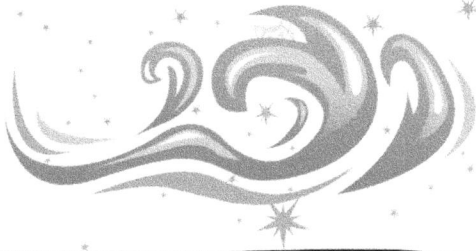

Rage Create

DATE ………… / ………… / 20 …………

I am always doing what I cannot do yet,
in order to learn how to do it.
– Vincent Van Gogh

BG:

Breath of Life

Close your eyes and breathe deeply for as long as possible.

Current Mood: Duration:

Sweet-Ass Affirmations

I am....

What are the two **most valuable actions** I will take today to progress toward my goals, dreams, and optimal health?

1.

2.

What makes me ☺ and why?

Wildcard

Knowledge Bomb

Ask your doctor to write a letter alerting the TSA to your diabetes and your need to carry medications, test strips, and other supplies if you fly on airplanes.

Sweet-Ass Reward

How will I reward myself after accomplishing my two valuable actions today?

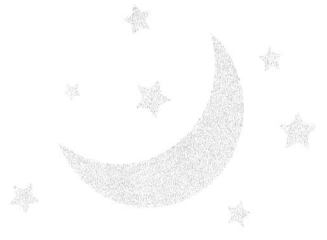

My **wins** for the day are:

Breath of Life

Close your eyes and breathe deeply for as long as possible.

Current Mood: Duration:

What are the two **most valuable actions** I will take tomorrow to
progress toward my goals, dreams, and optimal health?

1.

2.

Sweet-Ass Affirmations

I am....

Reflection and Thoughts

You are   41 % done with optimizing your diabetic lifestyle. ☺

BG:

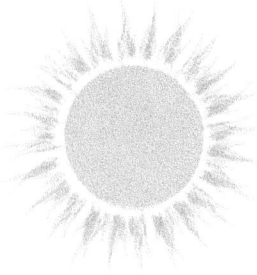

DATE .... / .... / 20 ....

There is a voice that doesn't use words. Listen.
– Rumi

BG:

Breath of Life

Close your eyes and breathe deeply for as long as possible.

Current Mood: Duration:

Sweet-Ass Affirmations

I am....

What are the two **most valuable actions** I will take today to progress toward my goals, dreams, and optimal health?

1.

2.

What makes me ☺ and why?

Wildcard

Knowledge Bomb

People should be nice to diabetics. We have to deal with pricks every day.

Sweet-Ass Reward

How will I reward myself after accomplishing my two valuable actions today?

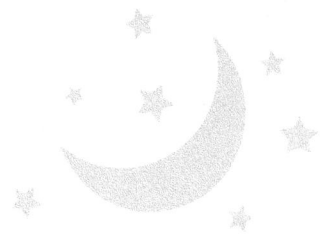

My **wins** for the day are:

Party Checklist

☐ Rx ☐ Test ☐ Water

☐ Nutrition ☐ Movement ☐ Reward

Breath of Life

Close your eyes and breathe deeply for as long as possible.

Current Mood: Duration:

What are the two **most valuable actions** I will take tomorrow to progress toward my goals, dreams, and optimal health?

1.

2.

Sweet-Ass Affirmations

I am....

Reflection and Thoughts

Wildcard: Experience Challenges

There is nothing more exciting than experiencing new things in life. Experience is the best form of education. No matter how much information you study or digest, nothing in life will have an impact on your journey more than experiences.

We realize experiencing new things can be uncomfortable. It's not easy to break our normal routines and try something different. However, it's nearly impossible to expand and grow without partaking in new adventures, experiences, and environments.

The good news: It's incredibly fun and transcendental to create new experiences in life. You will encounter so many people, places, and supportive energies that will help guide you along your journey.

Starting today, and randomly throughout the rest of the journal, you will notice several challenges in the wildcard box. Embrace these challenges as opportunities for growth. They aren't terrifying, daunting, or even hard. We have simply implied challenges, paired with ideas for experiences, to help you crack open your normal routine and grow within your journey.

We know you will have a blast. :)

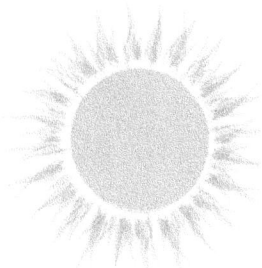

DATE .... / .... / 20 ....

If we were meant to stay in one place,
we'd have roots instead of feet.
– Rachel Wolchin

BG:

Breath of Life

Close your eyes and breathe deeply for as long as possible.

Current Mood: Duration:

Sweet-Ass Affirmations

I am....

What are the two **most valuable actions** I will take today to progress toward my goals, dreams, and optimal health?

1.

2.

What makes me ☺ and why?

Wildcard

Nature Challenge

Mother nature helps detox negative energy and stress. Plan a day trip to explore a natural landscape and connect with the healing powers of Earth.

Take a video and tag us
@partylikeadiabetic
for a chance to win swag.

Sweet-Ass Reward

How will I reward myself after accomplishing my two valuable actions today?

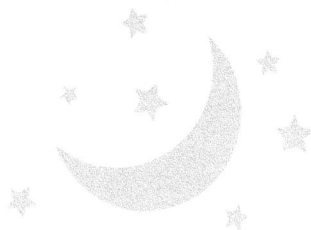

My **wins** for the day are:

Party Checklist

☐ Rx   ☐ Test   ☐ Water

☐ Nutrition   ☐ Movement   ☐ Reward

Breath of Life

Close your eyes and breathe deeply for as long as possible.

Current Mood: Duration:

What are the two **most valuable actions** I will take tomorrow to
progress toward my goals, dreams, and optimal health?

1.

2.

Sweet-Ass Affirmations

I am....

Reflection and Thoughts

You are   43 % done with optimizing your diabetic lifestyle. ☺   **BG:**

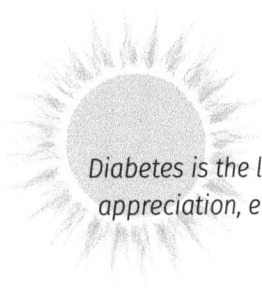

DATE .... / .... / 20 ....

Diabetes is the leading cause of courage, self-awareness, persistence, maturity, empathy, appreciation, enlightenment, understanding, compassion, bravery, fortitude, substance, personality, daring, grit, and guts.
– Unknown

BG:

Breath of Life

Close your eyes and breathe deeply for as long as possible.

Current Mood: Duration:

Sweet-Ass Affirmations

I am....

What are the two **most valuable actions** I will take today to progress toward my goals, dreams, and optimal health?

1.

2.

What makes me ☺ and why?

Wildcard

Knowledge Bomb

If you will be away from running water, bring alcohol wipes to clean your fingers before testing your blood sugar.

Sweet-Ass Reward

How will I reward myself after accomplishing my two valuable actions today?

My **wins** for the day are:

Party Checklist

☐ Rx ☐ Test ☐ Water

☐ Nutrition ☐ Movement ☐ Reward

Breath of Life

Close your eyes and breathe deeply for as long as possible.

Current Mood: Duration:

What are the two **most valuable actions** I will take tomorrow to progress toward my goals, dreams, and optimal health?

1.

2.

Sweet-Ass Affirmations

I am....

Reflection and Thoughts

You are 44 % done with optimizing your diabetic lifestyle. ☺

BG:

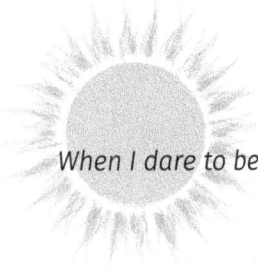

DATE .... / .... / 20 ....

When I dare to be powerful, to use my strength in the service of my vision, then it becomes less and less important whether I am afraid.
– Audrey Lorde

BG:

Breath of Life

Close your eyes and breathe deeply for as long as possible.

Current Mood: Duration:

Sweet-Ass Affirmations

I am....

What are the two **most valuable actions** I will take today to progress toward my goals, dreams, and optimal health?

1.

2.

What makes me ☺ and why?

Wildcard

A Letter to Diabetes

Take some time and go to your sacred space. Write a letter to your diabetes. What do you want to share, say, or explore?

Sweet-Ass Reward

How will I reward myself after accomplishing my two valuable actions today?

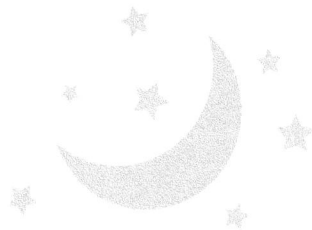

My **wins** for the day are:

Party Checklist

☐ Rx ☐ Test ☐ Water
☐ Nutrition ☐ Movement ☐ Reward

Breath of Life

Close your eyes and breathe deeply for as long as possible.

Current Mood: Duration:

What are the two **most valuable actions** I will take tomorrow to progress toward my goals, dreams, and optimal health?

1.

2.

Sweet-Ass Affirmations

I am....

Reflection and Thoughts

You are 45 % done with optimizing your diabetic lifestyle. ☺

BG:

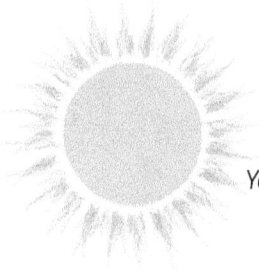

DATE .... / .... / 20 ....

You create opportunities by performing, not complaining.
– Muriel Siebert

BG:

Breath of Life

Close your eyes and breathe deeply for as long as possible.

Current Mood: Duration:

Sweet-Ass Affirmations

I am....

What are the two **most valuable actions** I will take today to progress toward my goals, dreams, and optimal health?

1.

2.

What makes me ☺ and why?

Wildcard

Knowledge Bomb

You may have diabetes, but diabetes does not have you.

Sweet-Ass Reward

How will I reward myself after accomplishing my two valuable actions today?

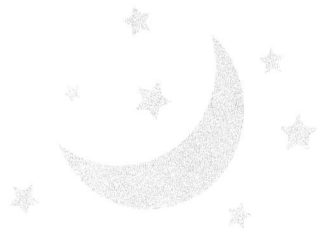

My **wins** for the day are:

Party Checklist

☐ Rx   ☐ Test   ☐ Water
☐ Nutrition   ☐ Movement   ☐ Reward

Breath of Life

Close your eyes and breathe deeply for as long as possible.

Current Mood: Duration:

What are the two **most valuable actions** I will take tomorrow to
progress toward my goals, dreams, and optimal health?

1.

2.

Sweet-Ass Affirmations

I am....

Reflection and Thoughts

You are   46 % done with optimizing your diabetic lifestyle. ☺   **BG:**

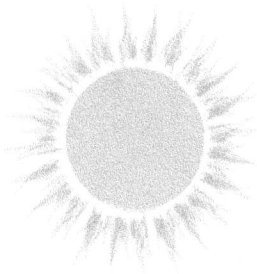

DATE .... / .... / 20 ....

Authenticity happens when your love of truth becomes
more important than your need for approval.
– Unknown

BG:

Breath of Life

Close your eyes and breathe deeply for as long as possible.

Current Mood: Duration:

Sweet-Ass Affirmations

I am....

What are the two **most valuable actions** I will take today to progress toward my goals, dreams, and optimal health?

1.

2.

What makes me ☺ and why?

Wildcard

Knowledge Bomb

Diabetics are naturally sweet.

Sweet-Ass Reward

How will I reward myself after accomplishing my two valuable actions today?

My **wins** for the day are:

Party Checklist

☐ Rx ☐ Test ☐ Water

☐ Nutrition ☐ Movement ☐ Reward

Breath of Life

Close your eyes and breathe deeply for as long as possible.

Current Mood: Duration:

What are the two **most valuable actions** I will take tomorrow to progress toward my goals, dreams, and optimal health?

1.

2.

Sweet-Ass Affirmations

I am....

Reflection and Thoughts

You are 47 % done with optimizing your diabetic lifestyle. ☺

BG:

DATE .... / .... / 20 ....

I believe in God, only I spell it Nature.
– Frank Lloyd Wright

BG:

Breath of Life

Close your eyes and breathe deeply for as long as possible.

Current Mood: Duration:

Sweet-Ass Affirmations

I am....

What are the two **most valuable actions** I will take today to progress toward my goals, dreams, and optimal health?

1.

2.

What makes me ☺ and why?

Wildcard

Meal Magic

Have you explored prepping your meals at the beginning of the week? Not only is it convenient, but it ensures you are getting proper nutrition and more stable blood sugar levels.

Sweet-Ass Reward

How will I reward myself after accomplishing my two valuable actions today?

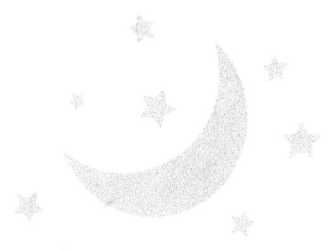

My **wins** for the day are:

Party Checklist

☐ Rx ☐ Test ☐ Water

☐ Nutrition ☐ Movement ☐ Reward

Breath of Life

Close your eyes and breathe deeply for as long as possible.

Current Mood: Duration:

What are the two **most valuable actions** I will take tomorrow to progress toward my goals, dreams, and optimal health?

1.

2.

Sweet-Ass Affirmations

I am....

Reflection and Thoughts

You are 48 % done with optimizing your diabetic lifestyle. ☺

BG:

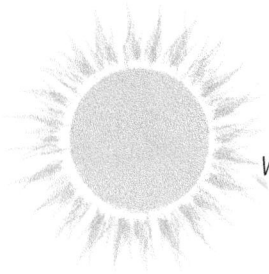

DATE .... / .... / 20 ....

*We are so successful at being comfortable, that comfort
has become the enemy of our success.*
– Wim Hof

BG:

Breath of Life

Close your eyes and breathe deeply for as long as possible.

Current Mood: Duration:

Sweet-Ass Affirmations

I am....

What are the two **most valuable actions** I will take today to progress toward my goals, dreams, and optimal health?

1.

2.

What makes me ☺ and why?

Wildcard

Cold Shower Challenge

Turn your shower temperature down to cold for the last 45 seconds today. Cold showers improve circulation and immunity, reduce stress levels, and stimulate weight-loss, among many other benefits.

Sweet-Ass Reward

How will I reward myself after accomplishing my two valuable actions today?

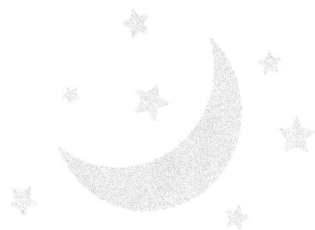

My **wins** for the day are:

Breath of Life

Close your eyes and breathe deeply for as long as possible.

Current Mood: Duration:

What are the two **most valuable actions** I will take tomorrow to progress toward my goals, dreams, and optimal health?

1.

2.

Sweet-Ass Affirmations

I am....

Reflection and Thoughts

You are   49 % done with optimizing your diabetic lifestyle. ☺

BG:

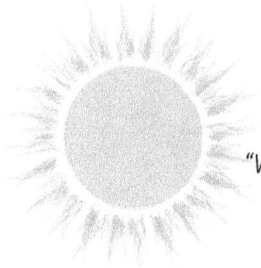

DATE .... / .... / 20 ....

"What day is it?" asked Pooh. "It's today," squeaked Piglet.
"My favorite day," said Pooh.
– A.A. Milne

BG:

Breath of Life

Close your eyes and breathe deeply for as long as possible.

Current Mood: Duration:

Sweet-Ass Affirmations

I am....

What are the two **most valuable actions** I will take today to progress toward my goals, dreams, and optimal health?

1.

2.

What makes me ☺ and why?

Wildcard

Knowledge Bomb

Seek healthy ways to cope with diabetes distress or burnout.

Check out some ideas in the bonus material at:
www.sweetassjournal.com/pladbonus

Sweet-Ass Reward

How will I reward myself after accomplishing my two valuable actions today?

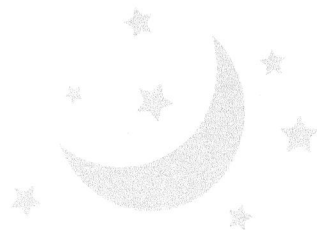

My **wins** for the day are:

Breath of Life

Close your eyes and breathe deeply for as long as possible.

Current Mood: Duration:

What are the two **most valuable actions** I will take tomorrow to progress toward my goals, dreams, and optimal health?

1.

2.

Sweet-Ass Affirmations

I am....

Reflection and Thoughts

You are **50** % done with optimizing your diabetic lifestyle. ☺

BG:

Sweet-Ass 100-Day Visions: Quarterly Review

Congrats, Wizard! You have made it through the first 50 days of journaling, which means you are halfway done with developing your optimal happiness and diabetic lifestyle.

As you did in your last quarter, it's time to review the progress and relevance of your visions!

Below, take a moment to write out your three updated visions. Remember to write them in the present or past tense, as if you are achieving or have already achieved them!

My sweet-ass visions are:

- ....
- ....
- ....

As you sow, so shall you reap. Everything you desire is on its way to you at warp speed!

Join our Patreon Community!
Eazy. Breezy. Diabeezy!

You are half-way through your 100 days! Have you joined our Patreon yet?

As we grow the Party Like A Diabetic community, we are also eternally grateful for your support and interaction. Just by purchasing this journal, you have helped expand our resources to reach new diabetics in need.

We have created an exclusive Patreon community and want to invite you to join and help grow this mission!

As a Patreon supporter, you will get access to the following:

- **Premium health tips, articles, and tools** about various topics for personal optimization
- **Live group/mastermind video calls** to engage with us and other members, including ongoing interviews with other authors, entrepreneurs, and medical experts
- **Community forum** where you can engage with other Diabadasses.
- **Exclusive bonus content**, including topics revolving around nutrition, diet planning, habit creation, happiness, exercise and more.
- **Discounts and early access** to new products (help us with beta testing!)
- **Meetups, parties, and local events** for our community!
- **Unlimited smiles**

We can't wait to party with you!

Join today: **www.sweetassjournal.com/pladpatreon**

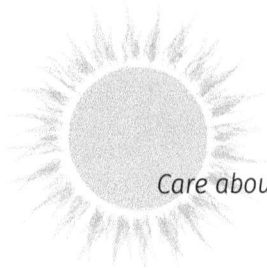

DATE ………… / ………… / 20 …………

Care about what other people think, and you will always be their prisoner.
– Lao Tzu

BG:

Breath of Life

Close your eyes and breathe deeply for as long as possible.

Current Mood: Duration:

Sweet-Ass Affirmations

I am….

What are the two **most valuable actions** I will take today to progress toward my goals, dreams, and optimal health?

1.

2.

What makes me 😊 and why?

Wildcard

Idea Muscle

Brainstorm a few ideas for relaxing your mind and body when you feel overwhelmed:

Sweet-Ass Reward

How will I reward myself after accomplishing my two valuable actions today?

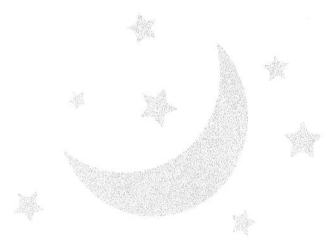

My **wins** for the day are:

Party Checklist

☐ Rx ☐ Test ☐ Water

☐ Nutrition ☐ Movement ☐ Reward

Breath of Life

Close your eyes and breathe deeply for as long as possible.

Current Mood: Duration:

What are the two **most valuable actions** I will take tomorrow to progress toward my goals, dreams, and optimal health?

1.

2.

Sweet-Ass Affirmations

I am....

Reflection and Thoughts

You are   51 % done with optimizing your diabetic lifestyle. ☺

BG:

DATE .... / .... / 20 ....

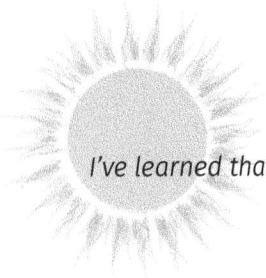

I've learned that people will forget what you said, people will forget what you did, but people will never forget how you made them feel.
– Maya Angelou

BG:

Breath of Life

Close your eyes and breathe deeply for as long as possible.

Current Mood: Duration:

Sweet-Ass Affirmations

I am....

What are the two **most valuable actions** I will take today to progress toward my goals, dreams, and optimal health?

1.

2.

What makes me ☺ and why?

Wildcard

Laughing Challenge

Force yourself to laugh loudly for 30 seconds. See what happens.... :)

Take a video and tag us @partylikeadiabetic for a chance to win swag.

Sweet-Ass Reward

How will I reward myself after accomplishing my two valuable actions today?

My **wins** for the day are:

Party Checklist

☐ Rx   ☐ Test   ☐ Water

☐ Nutrition   ☐ Movement   ☐ Reward

Breath of Life

Close your eyes and breathe deeply for as long as possible.

Current Mood: Duration:

What are the two **most valuable actions** I will take tomorrow to progress toward my goals, dreams, and optimal health?

1.

2.

Sweet-Ass Affirmations

I am....

Reflection and Thoughts

You are   52 % done with optimizing your diabetic lifestyle. ☺   **BG:**

Wildcard: 10-Day Minimalist Challenge — Removing Physical and Digital Distractions

We want to share something really simple, yet powerful with you:

You don't own your things; your things own you.

There is nothing wrong with having a relationship with material items, but how many of those material items are contributing absolute value to your dreams and optimal lifestyle?

When you have less stuff, you have fewer distractions. When you have fewer distractions, you awaken your awareness. When you are more aware, you pay attention to the areas of life that matter the most, like forming stronger relationships and engaging in higher levels of creativity.

As you form stronger relationships and engage in higher levels of creativity, and even combine the two, you continuously open new doors that lead directly to clarity, purpose, and meaning in life.

When you live your life with a clear intent, you will discover that the pursuit of happiness you dream of is not only possible, it's absolute.

Clear intent allows direct focus on creating purpose, value, and meaning, which is the only way to create true happiness and freedom. Other perks stem from being minimal, too, like eliminating the emotional and physical cost of all these things. These costs are much greater than you think.

When you have things, there are costs involved with taking care of, accessorizing, upgrading, updating, charging, storing, maintaining, worrying about, thinking about, dusting, cleaning, protecting and even replacing them. You are spending your time, money, energy, and brainpower to make sure all of the above are taken care of, leaving little time, money, energy, and brainpower for carving out and working toward the magnificent future and healthy lifestyle you desire and deserve!

Over the next 10 days (and as often as you wish afterward), we challenge you to a minimalist game to eliminate physical and digital distractions that are not in alignment with your optimal self.

You can do this alone, or partner up with a friend (more fun and more accountability). Each day, for 10 days, you will get rid of the number of items for whatever day you are on. For example: On day one, you get rid of one thing. On day two, you get rid of two more things. On day 10, you get rid of 10 more things! Yes, this may seem like it's too much, but you will discover you have way more stuff of little value to you than you ever imagined.

The first few days may seem easy, but you will face harder decisions to get rid of things you're attached to. This fear is totally normal, but we promise you, once you get rid of those 'hard' items, you will forget you ever had them. When you reach day 10, you may become so addicted that you keep going.

Remember, this challenge works great for physical *and* digital items. If you get stuck on the physical side, try cleaning out your old cell phone contacts, or removing all the games and apps on your phone that suck you into rabbit holes of distraction.

Whenever questioning an item's worth, simply ask yourself, "Does this contribute absolute value to my life?" If the answer is yes, keep it. If not, donate it, trash it, sell it, or send it off to someone who will find absolute value in it as a gift.

Your challenge begins today in the wildcard box!

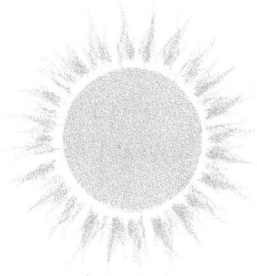

DATE .... / .... / 20 ....

Face it, accept it, deal with it, then let it go.
– Sheng Yen

BG:

Breath of Life

Close your eyes and breathe deeply for as long as possible.

Current Mood: Duration:

Sweet-Ass Affirmations

I am....

What are the two **most valuable actions** I will take today to progress toward my goals, dreams, and optimal health?

1.

2.

What makes me ☺ and why?

Wildcard

Minimalist Challenge Day 1

Get rid of one possession or distraction in your life that does not provide absolute value to your goals, dreams, and optimal health.

Sweet-Ass Reward

How will I reward myself after accomplishing my two valuable actions today?

My **wins** for the day are:

Party Checklist

☐ Rx   ☐ Test   ☐ Water
☐ Nutrition   ☐ Movement   ☐ Reward

Breath of Life

Close your eyes and breathe deeply for as long as possible.

Current Mood: Duration:

What are the two **most valuable actions** I will take tomorrow to
progress toward my goals, dreams, and optimal health?

1.

2.

Sweet-Ass Affirmations

I am....

Reflection and Thoughts

You are   53 % done with optimizing your diabetic lifestyle. ☺

BG:

DATE .... / .... / 20 ....

The ability to observe without evaluating
is the highest form of intelligence.
– Jiddu Krishnamurti

BG:

Breath of Life

Close your eyes and breathe deeply for as long as possible.

Current Mood: Duration:

Sweet-Ass Affirmations

I am....

What are the two **most valuable actions** I will take today to progress toward my goals, dreams, and optimal health?

1.

2.

What makes me ☺ and why?

Wildcard

Minimalist Challenge Day 2

Get rid of two possessions or distractions in your life that do not provide absolute value to your goals, dreams, and optimal health.

Sweet-Ass Reward

How will I reward myself after accomplishing my two valuable actions today?

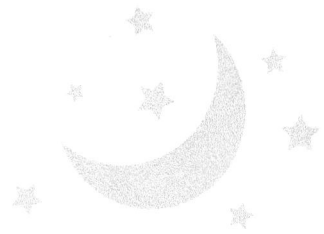

My **wins** for the day are:

Party Checklist

☐ Rx ☐ Test ☐ Water

☐ Nutrition ☐ Movement ☐ Reward

Breath of Life

Close your eyes and breathe deeply for as long as possible.

Current Mood: Duration:

What are the two **most valuable actions** I will take tomorrow to progress toward my goals, dreams, and optimal health?

1.

2.

Sweet-Ass Affirmations

I am....

Reflection and Thoughts

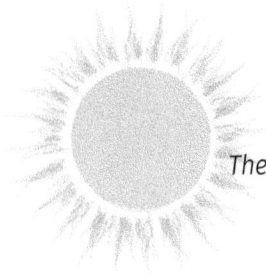

There are two mistakes one can make along the road to truth:
not going all the way, and not starting.
– Buddha

BG:

Breath of Life

Close your eyes and breathe deeply for as long as possible.

Current Mood: Duration:

Sweet-Ass Affirmations

I am....

What are the two **most valuable actions** I will take today to progress toward my goals, dreams, and optimal health?

1.

2.

What makes me ☺ and why?

Wildcard

Minimalist Challenge Day 3

Get rid of three possessions or distractions in your life that do not provide absolute value to your goals, dreams, and optimal health.

Sweet-Ass Reward

How will I reward myself after accomplishing my two valuable actions today?

My **wins** for the day are:

Party Checklist

☐ Rx ☐ Test ☐ Water

☐ Nutrition ☐ Movement ☐ Reward

Breath of Life

Close your eyes and breathe deeply for as long as possible.

Current Mood: Duration:

What are the two **most valuable actions** I will take tomorrow to progress toward my goals, dreams, and optimal health?

1.

2.

Sweet-Ass Affirmations

I am....

Reflection and Thoughts

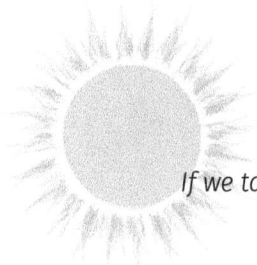

DATE .... / .... / 20 ....

If we take care of the minutes, the years will take care of themselves.
– Ben Franklin

BG:

Breath of Life

Close your eyes and breathe deeply for as long as possible.

Current Mood: Duration:

Sweet-Ass Affirmations

I am....

What are the two **most valuable actions** I will take today to progress toward my goals, dreams, and optimal health?

1.

2.

What makes me ☺ and why?

Wildcard

Minimalist Challenge Day 4

Get rid of four possessions or distractions in your life that do not provide absolute value to your goals, dreams, and optimal health.

Sweet-Ass Reward

How will I reward myself after accomplishing my two valuable actions today?

My **wins** for the day are:

Party Checklist

☐ Rx   ☐ Test   ☐ Water
☐ Nutrition   ☐ Movement   ☐ Reward

Breath of Life

Close your eyes and breathe deeply for as long as possible.

Current Mood: Duration:

What are the two **most valuable actions** I will take tomorrow to
progress toward my goals, dreams, and optimal health?

1.

2.

Sweet-Ass Affirmations

I am....

Reflection and Thoughts

You are   **56** % done with optimizing your diabetic lifestyle. ☺

BG:

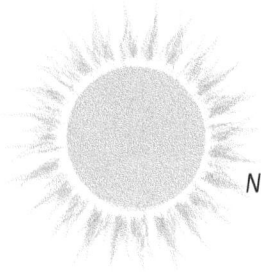

DATE .... / .... / 20 ....

Nobody achieves anything great by being happy and cozy.
– Alex Honnold

BG:

Breath of Life

Close your eyes and breathe deeply for as long as possible.

Current Mood: Duration:

Sweet-Ass Affirmations

I am....

What are the two **most valuable actions** I will take today to progress toward my goals, dreams, and optimal health?

1.

2.

What makes me ☺ and why?

Wildcard

Minimalist Challenge Day 5

Get rid of five possessions or distractions in your life that do not provide absolute value to your goals, dreams, and optimal health.

Sweet-Ass Reward

How will I reward myself after accomplishing my two valuable actions today?

My **wins** for the day are:

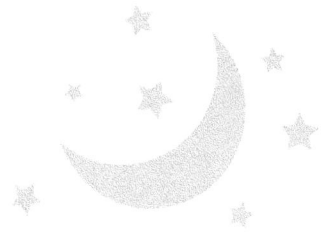

Breath of Life

Close your eyes and breathe deeply for as long as possible.

Current Mood: Duration:

What are the two **most valuable actions** I will take tomorrow to progress toward my goals, dreams, and optimal health?

1.

2.

Sweet-Ass Affirmations

I am....

Reflection and Thoughts

You are   **57** % done with optimizing your diabetic lifestyle. ☺

BG:

You can't see the label of the jar you are in.
– Valerie Groth

BG:

Breath of Life

Close your eyes and breathe deeply for as long as possible.

Current Mood: Duration:

Sweet-Ass Affirmations

I am....

What are the two **most valuable actions** I will take today to progress toward my goals, dreams, and optimal health?

1.

2.

What makes me ☺ and why?

Wildcard

Minimalist Challenge Day 6

Get rid of six possessions or distractions in your life that do not provide absolute value to your goals, dreams, and optimal health.

Sweet-Ass Reward

How will I reward myself after accomplishing my two valuable actions today?

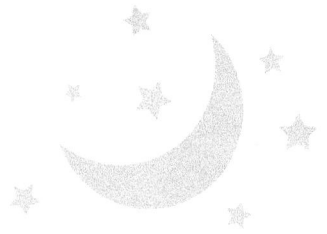

My **wins** for the day are:

Party Checklist

☐ Rx ☐ Test ☐ Water

☐ Nutrition ☐ Movement ☐ Reward

Breath of Life

Close your eyes and breathe deeply for as long as possible.

Current Mood: Duration:

What are the two **most valuable actions** I will take tomorrow to progress toward my goals, dreams, and optimal health?

1.

2.

Sweet-Ass Affirmations

I am....

Reflection and Thoughts

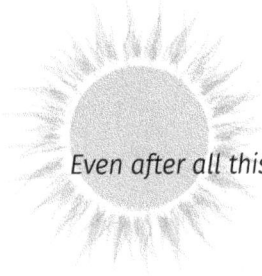

DATE .... / .... / 20 ....

Even after all this time, the Sun never says to the Earth, 'You owe me.' Look what happens
with a love like that, It lights up the whole sky.
– Interpretation from a Hafiz poem

BG:

Breath of Life

Close your eyes and breathe deeply for as long as possible.

Current Mood: Duration:

Sweet-Ass Affirmations

I am....

What are the two **most valuable actions** I will take today to progress toward my goals, dreams, and optimal health?

1.

2.

What makes me ☺ and why?

Wildcard

Minimalist Challenge Day 7

Get rid of seven possessions or distractions in your life that do not provide absolute value to your goals, dreams, and optimal health.

Sweet-Ass Reward

How will I reward myself after accomplishing my two valuable actions today?

My **wins** for the day are:

Breath of Life

Close your eyes and breathe deeply for as long as possible.

Current Mood: Duration:

What are the two **most valuable actions** I will take tomorrow to progress toward my goals, dreams, and optimal health?

1.

2.

Sweet-Ass Affirmations

I am....

Reflection and Thoughts

You are **59** % done with optimizing your diabetic lifestyle. ☺

BG:

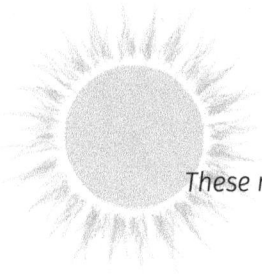

DATE .... / .... / 20 ....

These mountains you are carrying, you were only supposed to climb.
– Naswa Zebian

Breath of Life

Close your eyes and breathe deeply for as long as possible.

Current Mood: Duration:

Sweet-Ass Affirmations

I am....

What are the two **most valuable actions** I will take today to progress toward my goals, dreams, and optimal health?

1.

2.

What makes me ☺ and why?

Wildcard

Minimalist Challenge Day 8

Get rid of eight possessions or distractions in your life that do not provide absolute value to your goals, dreams, and optimal health.

Sweet-Ass Reward

How will I reward myself after accomplishing my two valuable actions today?

My **wins** for the day are:

Party Checklist

☐ Rx ☐ Test ☐ Water

☐ Nutrition ☐ Movement ☐ Reward

Breath of Life

Close your eyes and breathe deeply for as long as possible.

Current Mood: Duration:

What are the two **most valuable actions** I will take tomorrow to progress toward my goals, dreams, and optimal health?

1.

2.

Sweet-Ass Affirmations

I am....

Reflection and Thoughts

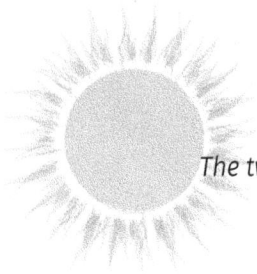

DATE   .... / .... / 20 ....

*The two most important days in your life are the day you are born
and the day you find out why.*
– Mark Twain

BG:

Breath of Life

Close your eyes and breathe deeply for as long as possible.

Current Mood: Duration:

Sweet-Ass Affirmations

I am....

What are the two **most valuable actions** I will take today to progress toward my goals, dreams, and optimal health?

1.

2.

What makes me ☺ and why?

Wildcard

Minimalist Challenge Day 9

Get rid of nine possessions or distractions in your life that do not provide absolute value to your goals, dreams, and optimal health.

Sweet-Ass Reward

How will I reward myself after accomplishing my two valuable actions today?

My **wins** for the day are:

Party Checklist

☐ Rx ☐ Test ☐ Water

☐ Nutrition ☐ Movement ☐ Reward

Breath of Life

Close your eyes and breathe deeply for as long as possible.

Current Mood: Duration:

What are the two **most valuable actions** I will take tomorrow to progress toward my goals, dreams, and optimal health?

1.

2.

Sweet-Ass Affirmations

I am....

Reflection and Thoughts

DATE .... / .... / 20 ....

You were wild once. Don't let them tame you.
– Isadora Duncan

BG:

Breath of Life

Close your eyes and breathe deeply for as long as possible.

Current Mood: Duration:

Sweet-Ass Affirmations

I am....

What are the two **most valuable actions** I will take today to progress toward my goals, dreams, and optimal health?

1.

2.

What makes me ☺ and why?

Wildcard

Minimalist Challenge Day 10

Get rid of ten possessions or distractions in your life that do not provide absolute value to your goals, dreams, and optimal health.

Sweet-Ass Reward

How will I reward myself after accomplishing my two valuable actions today?

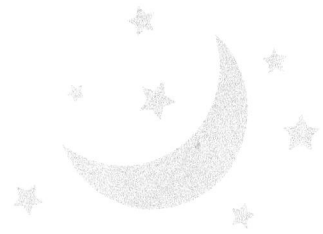

My **wins** for the day are:

Party Checklist

☐ Rx ☐ Test ☐ Water

☐ Nutrition ☐ Movement ☐ Reward

Breath of Life

Close your eyes and breathe deeply for as long as possible.

Current Mood: Duration:

What are the two **most valuable actions** I will take tomorrow to progress toward my goals, dreams, and optimal health?

1.

2.

Sweet-Ass Affirmations

I am....

Reflection and Thoughts

You are   62 % done with optimizing your diabetic lifestyle. ☺

BG:

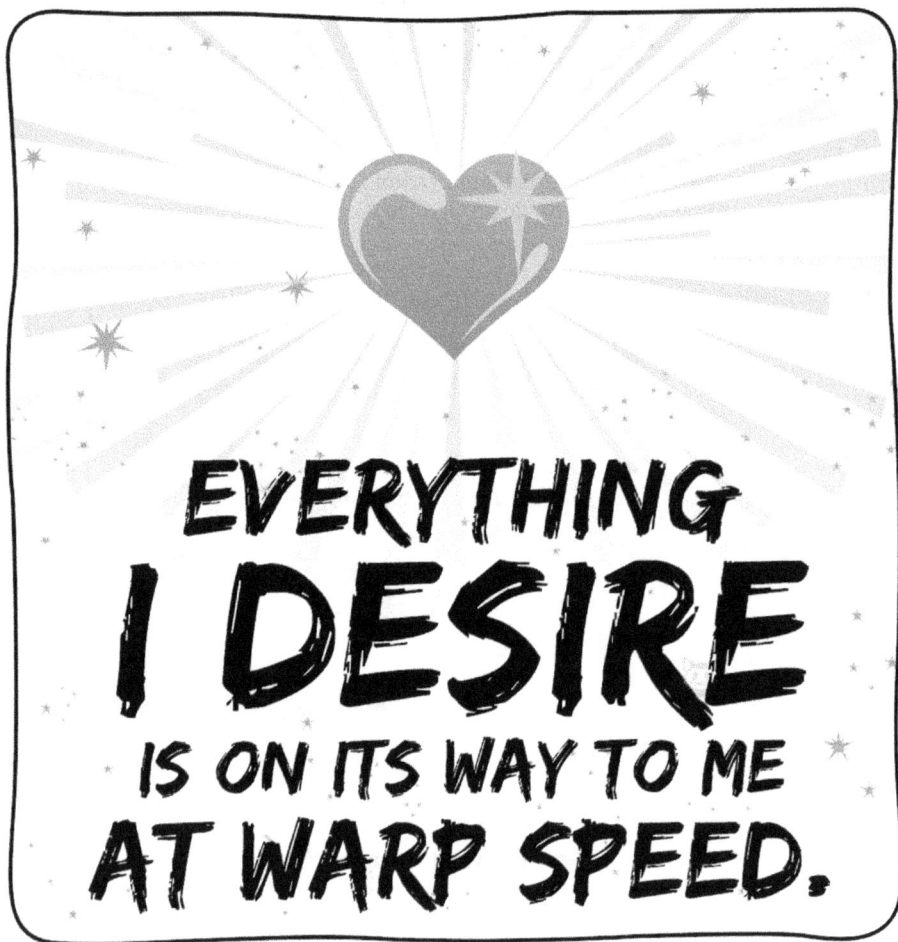

EVERYTHING **I DESIRE** IS ON ITS WAY TO ME AT WARP SPEED.

Ask the Universe for water and your
thirst will be quenched.
You are a magnet of your own blessings.
You know the essence of what you want
and you earn it. You are a fish in the water,
swimming in any direction you choose.
All visions that you support with your
highest intentions will come to pass.
Whatever you are reaching for, in return, is
reaching for you. Be one with your calling.

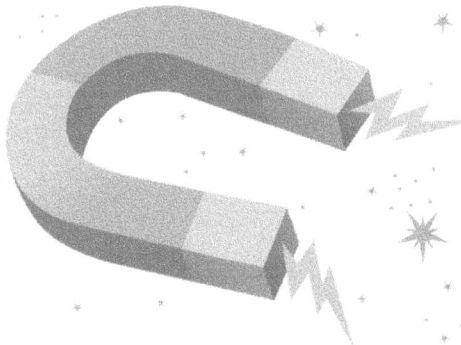

Rage Create

DATE .... / .... / 20 ....

Our truest life is when we are in dreams awake.
– Henry David Thoreau

BG:

Breath of Life

Close your eyes and breathe deeply for as long as possible.

Current Mood: Duration:

Sweet-Ass Affirmations

I am....

What are the two **most valuable actions** I will take today to progress toward my goals, dreams, and optimal health?

1.

2.

What makes me ☺ and why?

Wildcard

Meal Magic

Remember, drink 16 ounces of water when you wake up, 30 minutes before each meal, and before you go to sleep. Hydration fuels your health!

Sweet-Ass Reward

How will I reward myself after accomplishing my two valuable actions today?

My **wins** for the day are:

Party Checklist

☐ Rx   ☐ Test   ☐ Water

☐ Nutrition   ☐ Movement   ☐ Reward

Breath of Life

Close your eyes and breathe deeply for as long as possible.

Current Mood: Duration:

What are the two **most valuable actions** I will take tomorrow to
progress toward my goals, dreams, and optimal health?

1.

2.

Sweet-Ass Affirmations

I am....

Reflection and Thoughts

You are   63 % done with optimizing your diabetic lifestyle. ☺

BG:

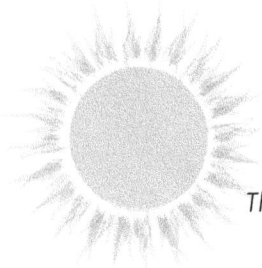

DATE .... / .... / 20 ....

We can easily forgive a child who is afraid of the dark.
The real tragedy in life is when men are afraid of the light.
– Plato

BG:

Breath of Life

Close your eyes and breathe deeply for as long as possible.

Current Mood: Duration:

Sweet-Ass Affirmations

I am....

What are the two **most valuable actions** I will take today to progress toward my goals, dreams, and optimal health?

1.

2.

What makes me 😊 and why?

Wildcard

Abundance List

I have an abundance of:

Sweet-Ass Reward

How will I reward myself after accomplishing my two valuable actions today?

My **wins** for the day are:

Party Checklist

☐ Rx ☐ Test ☐ Water

☐ Nutrition ☐ Movement ☐ Reward

Breath of Life

Close your eyes and breathe deeply for as long as possible.

Current Mood: Duration:

What are the two **most valuable actions** I will take tomorrow to progress toward my goals, dreams, and optimal health?

1.

2.

Sweet-Ass Affirmations

I am....

Reflection and Thoughts

You are 64 % done with optimizing your diabetic lifestyle. ☺

BG:

DATE .... / .... / 20 ....

We must be willing to let go of the life we planned
so as to have the life that is waiting for us.
– Joseph Campbell

BG:

Breath of Life

Close your eyes and breathe deeply for as long as possible.

Current Mood: Duration:

Sweet-Ass Affirmations

I am....

What are the two **most valuable actions** I will take today to progress toward my goals, dreams, and optimal health?

1.

2.

What makes me ☺ and why?

Sweet-Ass Reward

How will I reward myself after accomplishing my two valuable actions today?

Wildcard

Idea Muscle

List a few ideas for strengthening your diabetic support community:

My **wins** for the day are:

Party Checklist

☐ Rx ☐ Test ☐ Water

☐ Nutrition ☐ Movement ☐ Reward

Breath of Life

Close your eyes and breathe deeply for as long as possible.

Current Mood: Duration:

What are the two **most valuable actions** I will take tomorrow to
progress toward my goals, dreams, and optimal health?

1.

2.

Sweet-Ass Affirmations

I am....

Reflection and Thoughts

You are **65** % done with optimizing your diabetic lifestyle. ☺

BG:

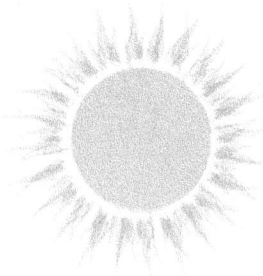

DATE ………… / ………… / 20 ……….

Remember no one can make you
feel inferior without your consent.
– Eleanor Roosevelt

BG:

Breath of Life

Close your eyes and breathe deeply for as long as possible.

Current Mood: Duration:

Sweet-Ass Affirmations

I am….

What are the two **most valuable actions** I will take today to progress toward my goals, dreams, and optimal health?

1.

2.

What makes me ☺ and why?

Wildcard

Electronic Ban Challenge

Turn off your cell phone, television, computer, and other electronics for a minimum two-hour uninterrupted period.

Sweet-Ass Reward

How will I reward myself after accomplishing my two valuable actions today?

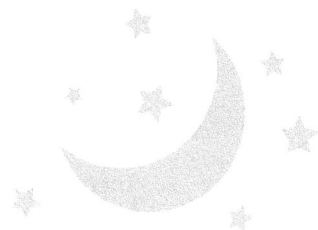

My **wins** for the day are:

Party Checklist

☐ Rx ☐ Test ☐ Water

☐ Nutrition ☐ Movement ☐ Reward

Breath of Life

Close your eyes and breathe deeply for as long as possible.

Current Mood: Duration:

What are the two **most valuable actions** I will take tomorrow to progress toward my goals, dreams, and optimal health?

1.

2.

Sweet-Ass Affirmations

I am....

Reflection and Thoughts

You are 66 % done with optimizing your diabetic lifestyle. ☺   **BG:**

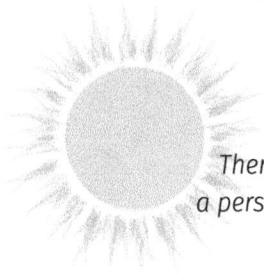

DATE .... / .... / 20 ....

There is absolutely nothing in this world more irresistible than
a person who inspires by simply wearing their soul on their sleeve.
— Christopher Poindexter

BG:

Breath of Life

Close your eyes and breathe deeply for as long as possible.

Current Mood: Duration:

Sweet-Ass Affirmations

I am....

What are the two **most valuable actions** I will take today to progress toward my goals, dreams, and optimal health?

1.

2.

What makes me ☺ and why?

Wildcard

Giving Challenge

What will I give today to impact someone's life in a positive way?

Sweet-Ass Reward

How will I reward myself after accomplishing my two valuable actions today?

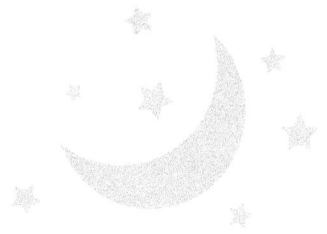

My **wins** for the day are:

Party Checklist

☐ Rx   ☐ Test   ☐ Water

☐ Nutrition   ☐ Movement   ☐ Reward

Breath of Life

Close your eyes and breathe deeply for as long as possible.

Current Mood: Duration:

What are the two **most valuable actions** I will take tomorrow to
progress toward my goals, dreams, and optimal health?

1.

2.

Sweet-Ass Affirmations

I am....

Reflection and Thoughts

You are   **67** % done with optimizing your diabetic lifestyle. ☺   **BG:**

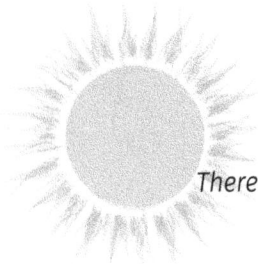

DATE .... / .... / 20 ....

There is no greater agony than bearing an untold story inside you.
— Maya Angelou

BG:

Breath of Life

Close your eyes and breathe deeply for as long as possible.

Current Mood:

Duration:

Sweet-Ass Affirmations

I am....

What are the two **most valuable actions** I will take today to progress toward my goals, dreams, and optimal health?

1.

2.

What makes me ☺ and why?

Wildcard

Knowledge Bomb

Celebrate YOU and all your hard work. Making the most out of your circumstance is powerful, respectful, and cultivates self love.

Sweet-Ass Reward

How will I reward myself after accomplishing my two valuable actions today?

My **wins** for the day are:

Party Checklist

☐ Rx ☐ Test ☐ Water

☐ Nutrition ☐ Movement ☐ Reward

Breath of Life

Close your eyes and breathe deeply for as long as possible.

Current Mood: Duration:

What are the two **most valuable actions** I will take tomorrow to progress toward my goals, dreams, and optimal health?

1.

2.

Sweet-Ass Affirmations

I am....

Reflection and Thoughts

You are **68** % done with optimizing your diabetic lifestyle. ☺   **BG:**

DATE .... / .... / 20 ....

It's hard to beat a person who never gives up.
– Babe Ruth

BG:

Breath of Life

Close your eyes and breathe deeply for as long as possible.

Current Mood: Duration:

Sweet-Ass Affirmations

I am....

What are the two **most valuable actions** I will take today to progress toward my goals, dreams, and optimal health?

1.

2.

What makes me ☺ and why?

Wildcard

Exercise / Movement

Have you moved that sexy body yet today? Choose a few exercises on your own or from the bonus material and get that blood flowing!

Sweet-Ass Reward

How will I reward myself after accomplishing my two valuable actions today?

My **wins** for the day are:

Party Checklist

☐ Rx   ☐ Test   ☐ Water

☐ Nutrition   ☐ Movement   ☐ Reward

Breath of Life

Close your eyes and breathe deeply for as long as possible.

Current Mood: Duration:

What are the two **most valuable actions** I will take tomorrow to progress toward my goals, dreams, and optimal health?

1.

2.

Sweet-Ass Affirmations

I am....

Reflection and Thoughts

You are **69** % done with optimizing your diabetic lifestyle. ☺

BG:

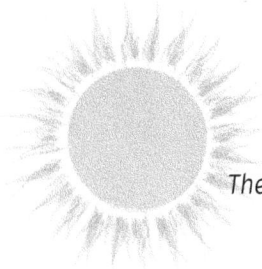

DATE .... / .... / 20 ....

The greatest gift you can give another is your own happiness.
– Esther Hicks

BG:

Breath of Life

Close your eyes and breathe deeply for as long as possible.

Current Mood: Duration:

Sweet-Ass Affirmations

I am....

What are the two **most valuable actions** I will take today to progress toward my goals, dreams, and optimal health?

1.

2.

What makes me ☺ and why?

Wildcard

Knowledge Bomb

Diabetes is hard, but you don't have to be hard on yourself.

Sweet-Ass Reward

How will I reward myself after accomplishing my two valuable actions today?

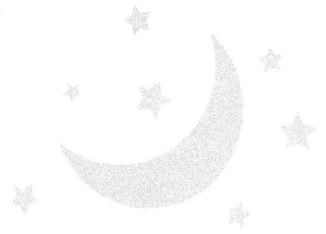

My **wins** for the day are:

Party Checklist

☐ Rx ☐ Test ☐ Water

☐ Nutrition ☐ Movement ☐ Reward

Breath of Life

Close your eyes and breathe deeply for as long as possible.

Current Mood: Duration:

What are the two **most valuable actions** I will take tomorrow to progress toward my goals, dreams, and optimal health?

1.

2.

Sweet-Ass Affirmations

I am....

Reflection and Thoughts

You are **70** % done with optimizing your diabetic lifestyle. ☺

BG:

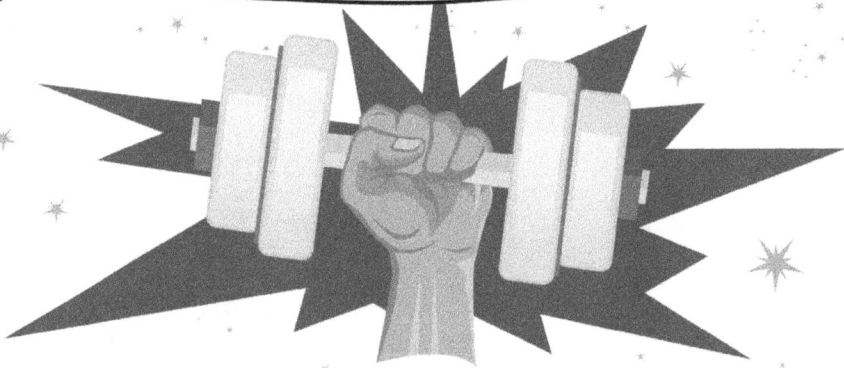

I FEED MY INNER PASSENGER **SUPERFOODS** OF STRENGTH, PROSPERITY, AND RESILIENCE. THEREFORE, I AM **STRONG, PROSPEROUS, AND RESILIENT.**

Inside every one of us is a beauty and a beast. The beauty is a product of our joy, peace, love, humility, generosity, and compassion. The beast is a product of our jealousy, arrogance, ego, greed, regret, and sorrow.
Feed the beauty and not the beast.

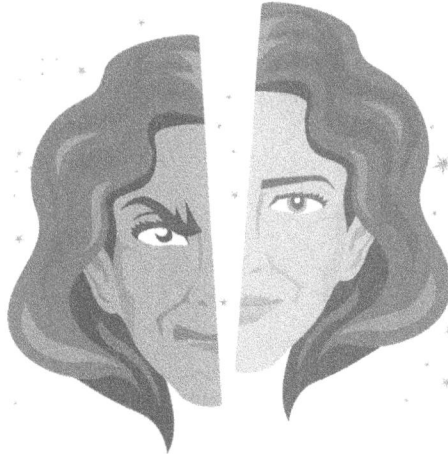

Rage Create

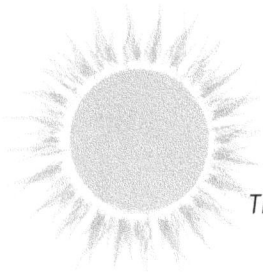

DATE .... / .... / 20 ....

Take your impossibilities and cradle them gently.
Then kiss 'em tenderly and throw them off a moving train.
– Alexander Franzen

BG:

Breath of Life

Close your eyes and breathe deeply for as long as possible.

Current Mood: Duration:

Sweet-Ass Affirmations

I am....

What are the two **most valuable actions** I will take today to progress toward my goals, dreams, and optimal health?

1.

2.

What makes me ☺ and why?

Wildcard

Knowledge Bomb

Well-managed diabetes is the leading cause of a long, happy, and healthy life.

Sweet-Ass Reward

How will I reward myself after accomplishing my two valuable actions today?

My **wins** for the day are:

Party Checklist

☐ Rx   ☐ Test   ☐ Water

☐ Nutrition   ☐ Movement   ☐ Reward

Breath of Life

Close your eyes and breathe deeply for as long as possible.

Current Mood: Duration:

What are the two **most valuable actions** I will take tomorrow to progress toward my goals, dreams, and optimal health?

1.

2.

Sweet-Ass Affirmations

I am....

Reflection and Thoughts

You are   **71**% done with optimizing your diabetic lifestyle. ☺

BG:

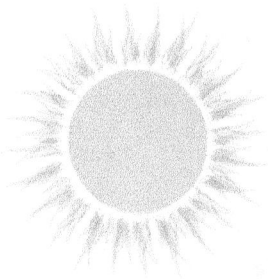

DATE .... / .... / 20 ....

*Do every act of your life as though it
were the very last act of your life.*
– Marcus Aurelius

BG:

Breath of Life

Close your eyes and breathe deeply for as long as possible.

Current Mood: Duration:

Sweet-Ass Affirmations

I am....

What are the two **most valuable actions** I will take today to progress toward my goals, dreams, and optimal health?

1.

2.

What makes me ☺ and why?

Wildcard

Sharing Challenge

Share your story of diabetes with an individual, group, or within your support system to help inspire others to embrace their health journey.

Sweet-Ass Reward

How will I reward myself after accomplishing my two valuable actions today?

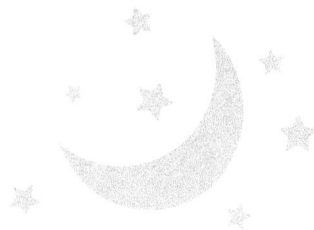

My **wins** for the day are:

Party Checklist

☐ Rx   ☐ Test   ☐ Water

☐ Nutrition   ☐ Movement   ☐ Reward

Breath of Life

Close your eyes and breathe deeply for as long as possible.

Current Mood: Duration:

What are the two **most valuable actions** I will take tomorrow to progress toward my goals, dreams, and optimal health?

1.

2.

Sweet-Ass Affirmations

I am....

Reflection and Thoughts

You are 72 % done with optimizing your diabetic lifestyle. ☺

BG:

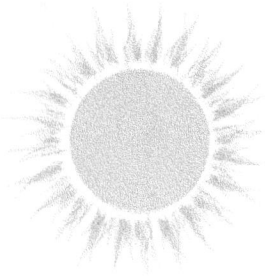

DATE .... / .... / 20 ....

Remember that not getting what you want is
sometimes a wonderful stroke of luck.
– Dalai Lama

BG:

Breath of Life

Close your eyes and breathe deeply for as long as possible.

Current Mood: Duration:

Sweet-Ass Affirmations

I am....

What are the two **most valuable actions** I will take today to progress toward my goals, dreams, and optimal health?

1.

2.

What makes me ☺ and why?

Wildcard

Abundance List

I have an abundance of:

Sweet-Ass Reward

How will I reward myself after accomplishing my two valuable actions today?

My **wins** for the day are:

Party Checklist

☐ Rx   ☐ Test   ☐ Water

☐ Nutrition   ☐ Movement   ☐ Reward

Breath of Life

Close your eyes and breathe deeply for as long as possible.

Current Mood: Duration:

What are the two **most valuable actions** I will take tomorrow to progress toward my goals, dreams, and optimal health?

1.

2.

Sweet-Ass Affirmations

I am....

Reflection and Thoughts

You are   73 % done with optimizing your diabetic lifestyle. ☺

BG:

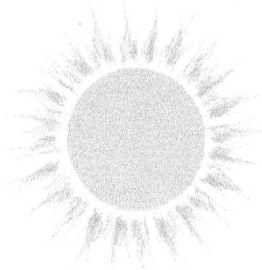

DATE .... / .... / 20 ....

Talent is a pursued interest. Anything you
are willing to practice, you can do.
– Bob Ross

BG:

Breath of Life

Close your eyes and breathe deeply for as long as possible.

Current Mood: Duration:

Sweet-Ass Affirmations

I am....

What are the two **most valuable actions** I will take today to progress toward my goals, dreams, and optimal health?

1.

2.

What makes me ☺ and why?

Wildcard

Giving Challenge

What will I give today to impact someone's life in a positive way?

Sweet-Ass Reward

How will I reward myself after accomplishing my two valuable actions today?

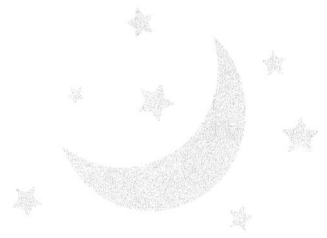

My **wins** for the day are:

Party Checklist

☐ Rx ☐ Test ☐ Water

☐ Nutrition ☐ Movement ☐ Reward

Breath of Life

Close your eyes and breathe deeply for as long as possible.

Current Mood: Duration:

What are the two **most valuable actions** I will take tomorrow to progress toward my goals, dreams, and optimal health?

1.

2.

Sweet-Ass Affirmations

I am....

Reflection and Thoughts

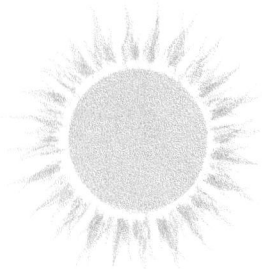

DATE .... / .... / 20 ....

The notes are right under your fingers. You just gotta'
take the time out to play the notes. That's life.
– Ray Charles

BG:

Breath of Life

Close your eyes and breathe deeply for as long as possible.

Current Mood: Duration:

Sweet-Ass Affirmations

I am....

What are the two **most valuable actions** I will take today to progress toward my goals, dreams, and optimal health?

1.

2.

What makes me ☺ and why?

Wildcard

Knowledge Bomb

Be your biggest advocate!

Sweet-Ass Reward

How will I reward myself after accomplishing my two valuable actions today?

My **wins** for the day are:

Party Checklist

☐ Rx   ☐ Test   ☐ Water

☐ Nutrition   ☐ Movement   ☐ Reward

Breath of Life

Close your eyes and breathe deeply for as long as possible.

Current Mood: Duration:

What are the two **most valuable actions** I will take tomorrow to progress toward my goals, dreams, and optimal health?

1.

2.

Sweet-Ass Affirmations

I am....

Reflection and Thoughts

You are   **75** % done with optimizing your diabetic lifestyle. ☺

BG:

Sweet-Ass 100-Day Visions: Quarterly Review

Party time! You have made it through the first 75 days of journaling, which means you are 75% done with developing your optimal happiness and diabetic lifestyle.

As you did in your last quarter, it's time to review the progress and relevance of your visions!

Below, take a moment to write out your three updated visions. Remember to write them in the present or past tense, as if you are achieving or have already achieved them!

My sweet-ass visions are:

- ....
- ....
- ....

As you sow, so shall you reap. Everything you desire is on its way to you at warp speed!

Join our Patreon Community!

Eazy. Breezy. Diabeezy!

Hey diabadass! Have you joined our Patreon community yet?

As we grow the Party Like A Diabetic community, we are also eternally grateful for your support and interaction. Just by purchasing this journal, you have helped expand our resources to reach new diabetics in need.

We have created an exclusive Patreon community and want to invite you to join and help grow this mission!

As a Patreon supporter, you will get access to the following:

- **Premium health tips, articles, and tools** about various topics for personal optimization
- **Live group/mastermind video calls** to engage with us and other members, including ongoing interviews with other authors, entrepreneurs, and medical experts
- **Community forum** where you can engage with other Diabadasses.
- **Exclusive bonus content**, including topics revolving around nutrition, diet planning, habit creation, happiness, exercise and more.
- **Discounts and early access** to new products (help us with beta testing!)
- **Meetups, parties, and local events** for our community!
- **Unlimited smiles**

We can't wait to party with you!

Join today: **www.sweetassjournal.com/pladpatreon**

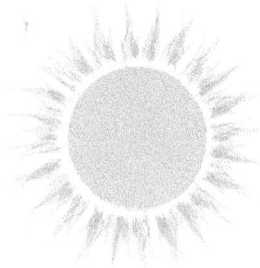

DATE .... / .... / 20 ....

Life isn't about waiting for the storm to pass.
It's about learning to dance in the rain.
– Vivian Greene

BG:

Breath of Life

Close your eyes and breathe deeply for as long as possible.

Current Mood: Duration:

Sweet-Ass Affirmations

I am....

What are the two **most valuable actions** I will take today to progress toward my goals, dreams, and optimal health?

1.

2.

What makes me ☺ and why?

Wildcard

Idea Muscle

Brainstorm a few ideas for taking yourself on a self-care date this week:

Sweet-Ass Reward

How will I reward myself after accomplishing my two valuable actions today?

My **wins** for the day are:

Party Checklist

☐ Rx   ☐ Test   ☐ Water

☐ Nutrition   ☐ Movement   ☐ Reward

Breath of Life

Close your eyes and breathe deeply for as long as possible.

Current Mood: Duration:

What are the two **most valuable actions** I will take tomorrow to progress toward my goals, dreams, and optimal health?

1.

2.

Sweet-Ass Affirmations

I am....

Reflection and Thoughts

You are   **76** % done with optimizing your diabetic lifestyle. ☺

BG:

DATE .... / .... / 20 ....

Believe you can and you're halfway there.
– Theodore Roosevelt

BG:

Breath of Life

Close your eyes and breathe deeply for as long as possible.

Current Mood: Duration:

Sweet-Ass Affirmations

I am....

What are the two **most valuable actions** I will take today to progress toward my goals, dreams, and optimal health?

1.

2.

What makes me 😊 and why?

Wildcard

Knowledge Bomb

Engage in "shared decision-making" with your doctor.

Sweet-Ass Reward

How will I reward myself after accomplishing my two valuable actions today?

My **wins** for the day are:

Breath of Life

Close your eyes and breathe deeply for as long as possible.

Current Mood: Duration:

What are the two **most valuable actions** I will take tomorrow to progress toward my goals, dreams, and optimal health?

1.

2.

Sweet-Ass Affirmations

I am....

Reflection and Thoughts

You are **77** % done with optimizing your diabetic lifestyle. ☺

BG:

DATE .... / .... / 20 ....

Live your life as if you have to live it over again.
– Heath Armstrong

BG:

Breath of Life

Close your eyes and breathe deeply for as long as possible.

Current Mood: Duration:

Sweet-Ass Affirmations

I am....

What are the two **most valuable actions** I will take today to progress toward my goals, dreams, and optimal health?

1.

2.

What makes me ☺ and why?

Wildcard

Knowledge Bomb

Write down all your questions and concerns before your doctor appointment to ensure they are addressed.

Sweet-Ass Reward

How will I reward myself after accomplishing my two valuable actions today?

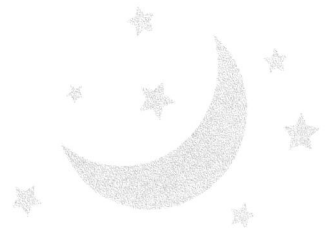

My **wins** for the day are:

Party Checklist

☐ Rx ☐ Test ☐ Water

☐ Nutrition ☐ Movement ☐ Reward

Breath of Life

Close your eyes and breathe deeply for as long as possible.

Current Mood: Duration:

What are the two **most valuable actions** I will take tomorrow to progress toward my goals, dreams, and optimal health?

1.

2.

Sweet-Ass Affirmations

I am....

Reflection and Thoughts

You are   78 % done with optimizing your diabetic lifestyle. ☺

BG:

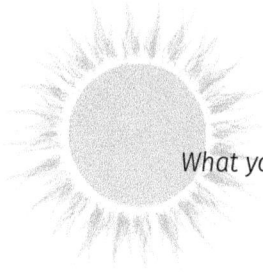

DATE .... / .... / 20 ....

What you do makes a difference, and you have to decide what kind of difference you want to make.
– Jane Goodall

BG:

Breath of Life

Close your eyes and breathe deeply for as long as possible.

Current Mood: Duration:

Sweet-Ass Affirmations

I am....

What are the two **most valuable actions** I will take today to progress toward my goals, dreams, and optimal health?

1.

2.

What makes me ☺ and why?

Wildcard

Appreciation Challenge

Reach out to someone you feel has supported you in your diabetic journey and let them know you appreciate them today.

Sweet-Ass Reward

How will I reward myself after accomplishing my two valuable actions today?

My **wins** for the day are:

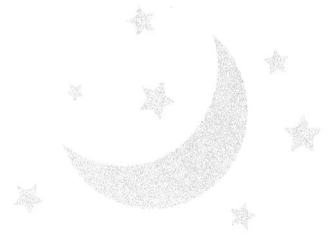

Party Checklist

☐ Rx   ☐ Test   ☐ Water

☐ Nutrition   ☐ Movement   ☐ Reward

Breath of Life

Close your eyes and breathe deeply for as long as possible.

Current Mood: Duration:

What are the two **most valuable actions** I will take tomorrow to progress toward my goals, dreams, and optimal health?

1.

2.

Sweet-Ass Affirmations

I am....

Reflection and Thoughts

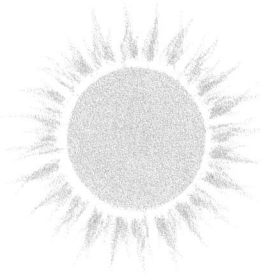

DATE .... / .... / 20 ....

Uncertainty is the gateway to possibility.
– Lissa Rankin

BG:

Breath of Life

Close your eyes and breathe deeply for as long as possible.

Current Mood: Duration:

Sweet-Ass Affirmations

I am....

What are the two **most valuable actions** I will take today to progress toward my goals, dreams, and optimal health?

1.

2.

What makes me ☺ and why?

Wildcard

Knowledge Bomb

Talk to your doctor about how to adjust your medications if you are crossing time zones.

Sweet-Ass Reward

How will I reward myself after accomplishing my two valuable actions today?

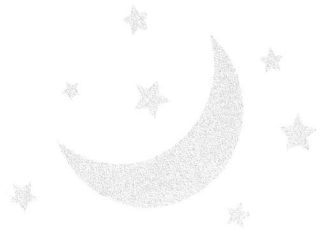

My **wins** for the day are:

Party Checklist

☐ Rx ☐ Test ☐ Water

☐ Nutrition ☐ Movement ☐ Reward

Breath of Life

Close your eyes and breathe deeply for as long as possible.

Current Mood: Duration:

What are the two **most valuable actions** I will take tomorrow to progress toward my goals, dreams, and optimal health?

1.

2.

Sweet-Ass Affirmations

I am....

Reflection and Thoughts

You are **80** % done with optimizing your diabetic lifestyle. ☺

BG:

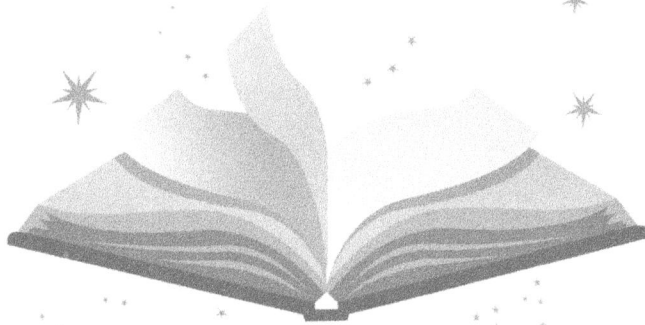

I CONTINUOUSLY PUSH
MYSELF TO LEARN
AND DEVELOP IN AREAS
OF LIFE THAT BRING ME
HAPPINESS, FREEDOM,
AND PURPOSE.

The definition of success is "the accomplishment of an aim or purpose." Success is extremely subjective and never guaranteed! However, if you do not try, you have a 100% chance of failing. Nothing ventured, nothing gained! Alternately, if you never stop trying, you have a 100% chance of learning and experiencing something new. If you commit to learning and gaining new experience in the direction of your dreams, you'll fill your journey with success, happiness, freedom and purpose.

Rage Create

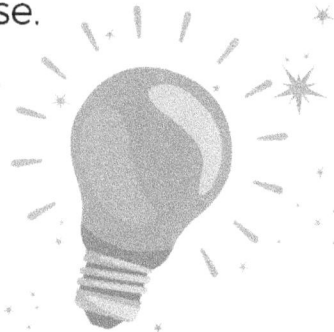

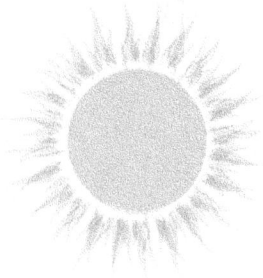

DATE .... / .... / 20 ....

Treat everyone you meet like God in drag.
– Ram Dass

BG:

Breath of Life

Close your eyes and breathe deeply for as long as possible.

Current Mood: Duration:

Sweet-Ass Affirmations

I am....

What are the two **most valuable actions** I will take today to progress toward my goals, dreams, and optimal health?

1.

2.

What makes me ☺ and why?

Wildcard

Knowledge Bomb

Lather on the SPF, as sunburns can increase blood sugars.

Sweet-Ass Reward

How will I reward myself after accomplishing my two valuable actions today?

My **wins** for the day are:

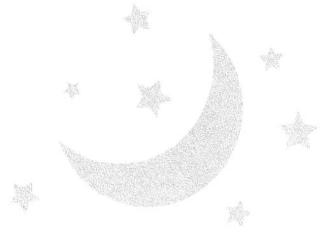

Breath of Life

Close your eyes and breathe deeply for as long as possible.

Current Mood: Duration:

What are the two **most valuable actions** I will take tomorrow to
progress toward my goals, dreams, and optimal health?

1.

2.

Sweet-Ass Affirmations

I am....

Reflection and Thoughts

You are **81** % done with optimizing your diabetic lifestyle. ☺   **BG:**

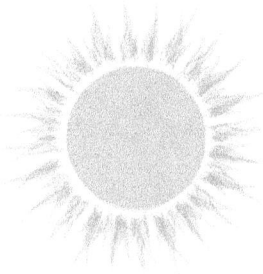

DATE .... / .... / 20 ....

Meditate, visualize, and create your own reality and the
universe will simply reflect back to you.
– Amit Ray

BG:

Breath of Life

Close your eyes and breathe deeply for as long as possible.

Current Mood: Duration:

Sweet-Ass Affirmations

I am....

What are the two **most valuable actions** I will take today to progress toward my goals, dreams, and optimal health?

1.

2.

What makes me ☺ and why?

Wildcard

Optimistic Challenge

Write down all the positive things you have learned from your diabetic journey.

Sweet-Ass Reward

How will I reward myself after accomplishing my two valuable actions today?

My **wins** for the day are:

Party Checklist

☐ Rx   ☐ Test   ☐ Water

☐ Nutrition   ☐ Movement   ☐ Reward

Breath of Life

Close your eyes and breathe deeply for as long as possible.

Current Mood: Duration:

What are the two **most valuable actions** I will take tomorrow to progress toward my goals, dreams, and optimal health?

1.

2.

Sweet-Ass Affirmations

I am....

Reflection and Thoughts

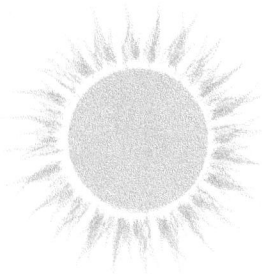

DATE .... / .... / 20 ....

Do not ruin today with mourning tomorrow.
– Catherynne M. Valente

BG:

Breath of Life

Close your eyes and breathe deeply for as long as possible.

Current Mood: Duration:

Sweet-Ass Affirmations

I am....

What are the two **most valuable actions** I will take today to progress toward my goals, dreams, and optimal health?

1.

2.

What makes me ☺ and why?

Wildcard

Meal Magic

Try not to add extra sugar to your meals, snacks, or drinks this week and see how it makes you feel. Also, notice the effect it has on your blood sugar.

Sweet-Ass Reward

How will I reward myself after accomplishing my two valuable actions today?

My **wins** for the day are:

Party Checklist

☐ Rx ☐ Test ☐ Water
☐ Nutrition ☐ Movement ☐ Reward

Breath of Life

Close your eyes and breathe deeply for as long as possible.

Current Mood: Duration:

What are the two **most valuable actions** I will take tomorrow to progress toward my goals, dreams, and optimal health?

1.

2.

Sweet-Ass Affirmations

I am....

Reflection and Thoughts

You are 83 % done with optimizing your diabetic lifestyle. ☺   **BG:**

DATE .... / .... / 20 ....

There is always a reason to complain, and always
a reason to dance. Choose to dance.
– Brad Montague

BG:

Breath of Life

Close your eyes and breathe deeply for as long as possible.

Current Mood: | Duration:

Sweet-Ass Affirmations

I am....

What are the two **most valuable actions** I will take today to progress toward my goals, dreams, and optimal health?

1.

2.

What makes me ☺ and why?

Wildcard

Giving Challenge

What will I give today to impact someone's life in a positive way?

Sweet-Ass Reward

How will I reward myself after accomplishing my two valuable actions today?

My **wins** for the day are:

Party Checklist

☐ Rx ☐ Test ☐ Water

☐ Nutrition ☐ Movement ☐ Reward

Breath of Life

Close your eyes and breathe deeply for as long as possible.

Current Mood: Duration:

What are the two **most valuable actions** I will take tomorrow to progress toward my goals, dreams, and optimal health?

1.

2.

Sweet-Ass Affirmations

I am....

Reflection and Thoughts

You are 84 % done with optimizing your diabetic lifestyle. ☺

BG:

DATE ………… / ………… / 20 …………

The creative adult is the child who survived.
– Ursula K. LeGuin

BG:

Breath of Life

Close your eyes and breathe deeply for as long as possible.

Current Mood: Duration:

Sweet-Ass Affirmations

I am....

What are the two **most valuable actions** I will take today to progress toward my goals, dreams, and optimal health?

1.

2.

What makes me ☺ and why?

Wildcard

Knowledge Bomb

It's okay to not be okay... okay?! :)

Sweet-Ass Reward

How will I reward myself after accomplishing my two valuable actions today?

My **wins** for the day are:

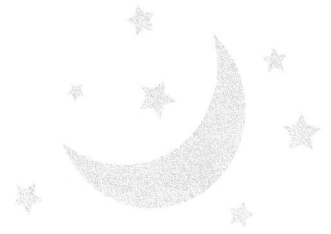

Party Checklist

☐ Rx   ☐ Test   ☐ Water

☐ Nutrition   ☐ Movement   ☐ Reward

Breath of Life

Close your eyes and breathe deeply for as long as possible.

Current Mood: Duration:

What are the two **most valuable actions** I will take tomorrow to progress toward my goals, dreams, and optimal health?

1.

2.

Sweet-Ass Affirmations

I am....

Reflection and Thoughts

You are   **85** % done with optimizing your diabetic lifestyle. ☺

BG:

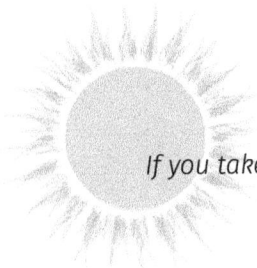

DATE ………… / ………… / 20 …………

If you take risks, you may fail. But if you don't take risks, you will surely fail.
The greatest risk of all is to do nothing.
– Robert Goizueta

BG:

Breath of Life

Close your eyes and breathe deeply for as long as possible.

Current Mood: Duration:

Sweet-Ass Affirmations

I am....

What are the two **most valuable actions** I will take today to progress toward my goals, dreams, and optimal health?

1.

2.

What makes me ☺ and why?

Sweet-Ass Reward

How will I reward myself after accomplishing my two valuable actions today?

Wildcard

Abundance List

I have an abundance of:

My **wins** for the day are:

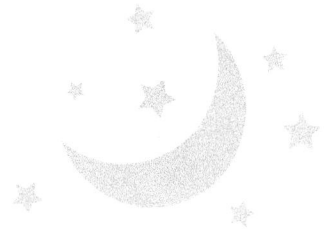

Party Checklist

☐ Rx ☐ Test ☐ Water

☐ Nutrition ☐ Movement ☐ Reward

Breath of Life

Close your eyes and breathe deeply for as long as possible.

Current Mood: Duration:

What are the two **most valuable actions** I will take tomorrow to progress toward my goals, dreams, and optimal health?

1.

2.

Sweet-Ass Affirmations

I am....

Reflection and Thoughts

You are **86** % done with optimizing your diabetic lifestyle. ☺

BG:

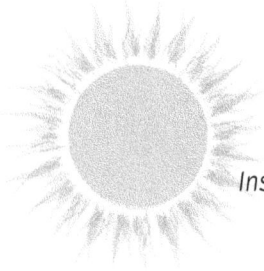

DATE ………… / ………… / 20 …………

Instead of holding yourself back, hold yourself accountable.
– Caitlin Grenier

BG:

Breath of Life

Close your eyes and breathe deeply for as long as possible.

Current Mood: Duration:

Sweet-Ass Affirmations

I am….

What are the two **most valuable actions** I will take today to progress toward my goals, dreams, and optimal health?

1.

2.

What makes me ☺ and why?

Wildcard

Exercise / Movement

Have you moved that sexy body yet today? Choose a few exercises on your own or from the bonus material and get that blood flowing!

Sweet-Ass Reward

How will I reward myself after accomplishing my two valuable actions today?

My **wins** for the day are:

Party Checklist

☐ Rx ☐ Test ☐ Water
☐ Nutrition ☐ Movement ☐ Reward

Breath of Life

Close your eyes and breathe deeply for as long as possible.

Current Mood: Duration:

What are the two **most valuable actions** I will take tomorrow to progress toward my goals, dreams, and optimal health?

1.

2.

Sweet-Ass Affirmations

I am....

Reflection and Thoughts

You are   **87** % done with optimizing your diabetic lifestyle. ☺   **BG:**

DATE .... / .... / 20 ....

I think we can make it. In fact I'm sure. And if you fall,
stand tall and come back for more.
– Tupac

BG:

Breath of Life

Close your eyes and breathe deeply for as long as possible.

Current Mood: Duration:

Sweet-Ass Affirmations

I am....

What are the two **most valuable actions** I will take today to progress toward my goals, dreams, and optimal health?

1.

2.

What makes me ☺ and why?

Wildcard

Order a New Journal!

You only have 12 days left in your 100-day journey! Make sure you order a fresh journal (for yourself and others you think would benefit) so you can keep your sweet-ass momentum!

Sweet-Ass Reward

How will I reward myself after accomplishing my two valuable actions today?

My **wins** for the day are:

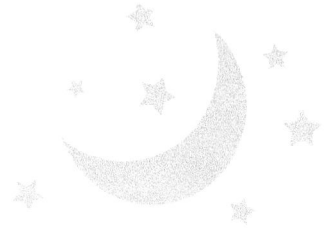

Party Checklist

☐ Rx   ☐ Test   ☐ Water

☐ Nutrition   ☐ Movement   ☐ Reward

Breath of Life

Close your eyes and breathe deeply for as long as possible.

Current Mood: Duration:

What are the two **most valuable actions** I will take tomorrow to progress toward my goals, dreams, and optimal health?

1.

2.

Sweet-Ass Affirmations

I am....

Reflection and Thoughts

You are **88** % done with optimizing your diabetic lifestyle. ☺

BG:

DATE .... / .... / 20 ....

Everything that irritates us about others can lead
to a deeper understanding of ourselves.
– Carl Jung

BG:

Breath of Life

Close your eyes and breathe deeply for as long as possible.

Current Mood: Duration:

Sweet-Ass Affirmations

I am....

What are the two **most valuable actions** I will take today to progress toward my goals, dreams, and optimal health?

1.

2.

What makes me ☺ and why?

Wildcard

Knowledge Bomb

Always pack more supplies than you think you will need while traveling. Having an excess is much better than running out!

Sweet-Ass Reward

How will I reward myself after accomplishing my two valuable actions today?

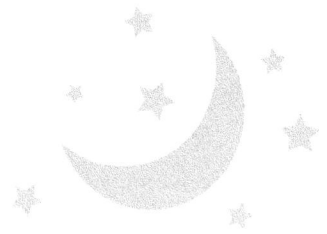

My **wins** for the day are:

Party Checklist

☐ Rx   ☐ Test   ☐ Water

☐ Nutrition   ☐ Movement   ☐ Reward

Breath of Life

Close your eyes and breathe deeply for as long as possible.

Current Mood: Duration:

What are the two **most valuable actions** I will take tomorrow to
progress toward my goals, dreams, and optimal health?

1.

2.

Sweet-Ass Affirmations

I am....

Reflection and Thoughts

You are **89**% done with optimizing your diabetic lifestyle. ☺   **BG:**

DATE .... / .... / 20 ....

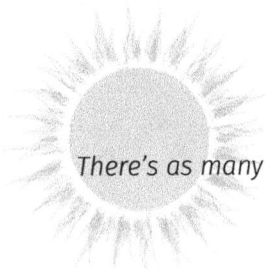

There's as many atoms in a single molecule of your DNA as there are stars in the typical galaxy. We are, each of us, a little universe.
– Neil deGrasse Tyson

BG:

Breath of Life

Close your eyes and breathe deeply for as long as possible.

Current Mood: Duration:

Sweet-Ass Affirmations

I am....

What are the two **most valuable actions** I will take today to progress toward my goals, dreams, and optimal health?

1.

2.

What makes me ☺ and why?

Wildcard

Knowledge Bomb

Exercise (even twerking) helps reduce insulin resistance (aka it helps insulin do its job!).

Sweet-Ass Reward

How will I reward myself after accomplishing my two valuable actions today?

My **wins** for the day are:

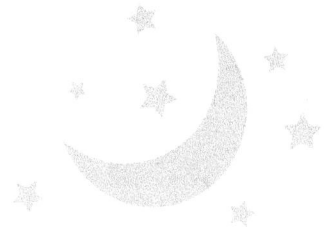

Party Checklist

☐ Rx ☐ Test ☐ Water

☐ Nutrition ☐ Movement ☐ Reward

Breath of Life

Close your eyes and breathe deeply for as long as possible.

Current Mood: Duration:

What are the two **most valuable actions** I will take tomorrow to progress toward my goals, dreams, and optimal health?

1.

2.

Sweet-Ass Affirmations

I am....

Reflection and Thoughts

You are **90** % done with optimizing your diabetic lifestyle. ☺

BG:

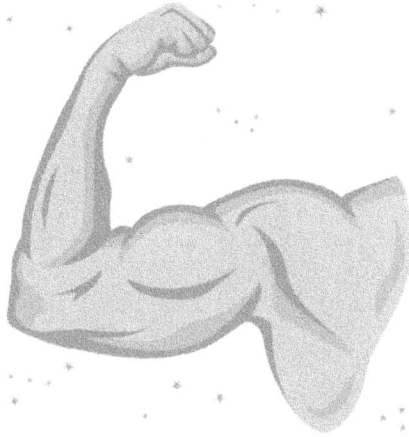

I EXERCISE
AND EXPAND MY
HAPPINESS MUSCLE
TO BEASTLY LEVELS
EVERY DAY.

It's easy to feel like happiness is elusive. You feel incredible and confident one day, and then unimportant, unattractive, and depressed the next. Before you know it, you end up slamming a bottle of wine and a tub of ice cream to help numb the gloom. But, just as people transition from unhealthy and overweight to healthy and fit, you can exercise your happiness muscle and build a life of smiles. With the tiniest practices of gratitude and mindfulness, and a focus on what truly lights you up, you can turn yourself into the Hulk Hogan of happiness. The army of sadness cannot break down your fortress if you are kicking their ass everyday.

Rage Create

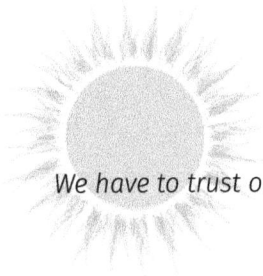

DATE .... / .... / 20 ....

We have to trust our instincts, honor them, and move forward despite what everybody says.
– Cynthia Miltenberger

BG:

Breath of Life

Close your eyes and breathe deeply for as long as possible.

Current Mood: Duration:

Sweet-Ass Affirmations

I am....

What are the two **most valuable actions** I will take today to progress toward my goals, dreams, and optimal health?

1.

2.

What makes me ☺ and why?

Wildcard

Early Riser Challenge

Set your alarm 30 minutes earlier and actually get up. Have a plan to do something extra or enjoy a little relaxation before your normal morning routine begins.

Sweet-Ass Reward

How will I reward myself after accomplishing my two valuable actions today?

My **wins** for the day are:

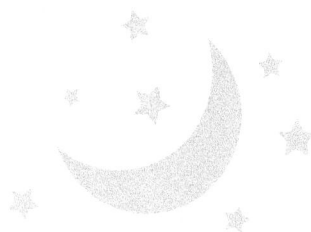

Party Checklist

☐ Rx ☐ Test ☐ Water

☐ Nutrition ☐ Movement ☐ Reward

Breath of Life

Close your eyes and breathe deeply for as long as possible.

Current Mood: Duration:

What are the two **most valuable actions** I will take tomorrow to progress toward my goals, dreams, and optimal health?

1.

2.

Sweet-Ass Affirmations

I am....

Reflection and Thoughts

You are **91**% done with optimizing your diabetic lifestyle. ☺

BG:

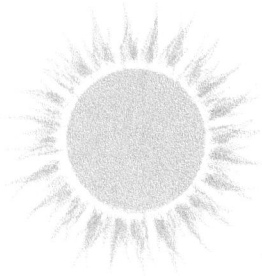

DATE .... / .... / 20 ....

A man who dares to waste one hour of life
has not discovered the value of life.
– Charles Darwin

BG:

Breath of Life

Close your eyes and breathe deeply for as long as possible.

Current Mood: Duration:

Sweet-Ass Affirmations

I am....

What are the two **most valuable actions** I will take today to progress toward my goals, dreams, and optimal health?

1.

2.

What makes me ☺ and why?

Wildcard

Idea Muscle

Brainstorm ideas for places you can go outside the light pollution of the city to look at the stars one night this week. You won't regret it.

Sweet-Ass Reward

How will I reward myself after accomplishing my two valuable actions today?

My **wins** for the day are:

Party Checklist

☐ Rx ☐ Test ☐ Water

☐ Nutrition ☐ Movement ☐ Reward

Breath of Life

Close your eyes and breathe deeply for as long as possible.

Current Mood: Duration:

What are the two **most valuable actions** I will take tomorrow to progress toward my goals, dreams, and optimal health?

1.

2.

Sweet-Ass Affirmations

I am....

Reflection and Thoughts

You are **92** % done with optimizing your diabetic lifestyle. ☺

BG:

DATE .... / .... / 20 ....

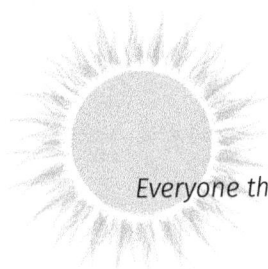

Everyone thinks of changing the world, but no one thinks of changing himself.
– Leo Tolstoy

BG:

Breath of Life

Close your eyes and breathe deeply for as long as possible.

Current Mood: Duration:

Sweet-Ass Affirmations

I am....

What are the two **most valuable actions** I will take today to progress toward my goals, dreams, and optimal health?

1.

2.

What makes me ☺ and why?

Wildcard

Knowledge Bomb

Foods that aren't likely to cause a big rise in your levels include sustainably farmed lean meat, poultry, fish, avocados, leafy vegetables, vegetables, eggs, and cheese.

Sweet-Ass Reward

How will I reward myself after accomplishing my two valuable actions today?

My **wins** for the day are:

Breath of Life

Close your eyes and breathe deeply for as long as possible.

Current Mood: Duration:

What are the two **most valuable actions** I will take tomorrow to progress toward my goals, dreams, and optimal health?

1.

2.

Sweet-Ass Affirmations

I am….

Reflection and Thoughts

You are **93** % done with optimizing your diabetic lifestyle. ☺

BG:

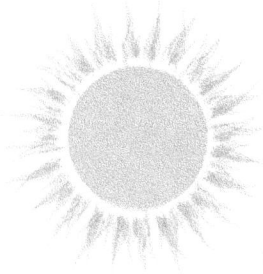

DATE .... / .... / 20 ....

Do not dwell in the past. Do not dream of the future.
Concentrate the mind on the present moment.
– Buddha

BG:

Breath of Life

Close your eyes and breathe deeply for as long as possible.

Current Mood: Duration:

Sweet-Ass Affirmations

I am....

What are the two **most valuable actions** I will take today to progress toward my goals, dreams, and optimal health?

1.

2.

What makes me ☺ and why?

Wildcard

Giving Challenge

What will I give today to impact someone's life in a positive way?

Sweet-Ass Reward

How will I reward myself after accomplishing my two valuable actions today?

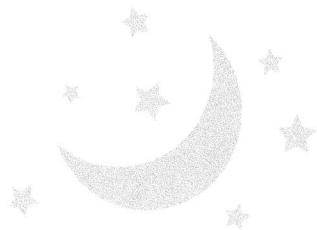

My **wins** for the day are:

Party Checklist

☐ Rx ☐ Test ☐ Water

☐ Nutrition ☐ Movement ☐ Reward

Breath of Life

Close your eyes and breathe deeply for as long as possible.

Current Mood: Duration:

What are the two **most valuable actions** I will take tomorrow to progress toward my goals, dreams, and optimal health?

1.

2.

Sweet-Ass Affirmations

I am....

Reflection and Thoughts

You are **94** % done with optimizing your diabetic lifestyle. ☺

BG:

DATE .... / .... / 20 ....

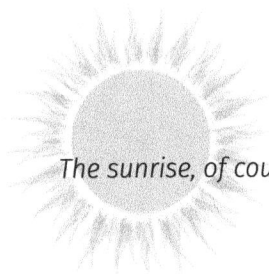

The sunrise, of course, doesn't care if we watch it or not. It will still keep on being beautiful, even if no one bothers to look at it.
– Gene Amole

BG:

Breath of Life

Close your eyes and breathe deeply for as long as possible.

Current Mood: Duration:

Sweet-Ass Affirmations

I am....

What are the two **most valuable actions** I will take today to progress toward my goals, dreams, and optimal health?

1.

2.

What makes me ☺ and why?

Wildcard

Knowledge Bomb

Having diabetes is NOT a personal failure. You are strong, beautiful, and full of resilience.

Sweet-Ass Reward

How will I reward myself after accomplishing my two valuable actions today?

My **wins** for the day are:

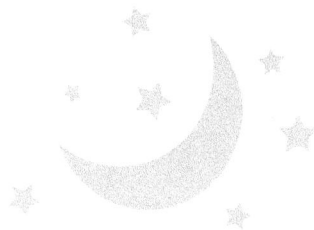

Party Checklist

☐ Rx ☐ Test ☐ Water

☐ Nutrition ☐ Movement ☐ Reward

Breath of Life

Close your eyes and breathe deeply for as long as possible.

Current Mood: Duration:

What are the two **most valuable actions** I will take tomorrow to progress toward my goals, dreams, and optimal health?

1.

2.

Sweet-Ass Affirmations

I am....

Reflection and Thoughts

You are **95** % done with optimizing your diabetic lifestyle. ☺

BG:

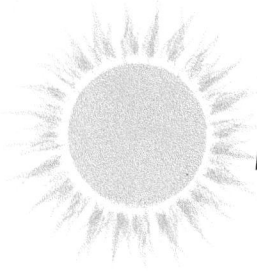

DATE .... / .... / 20 ....

Every single day of our life is a precious moment, and we
have no guarantees on how many of these we will have.
– Jeena Cho

BG:

Breath of Life

Close your eyes and breathe deeply for as long as possible.

Current Mood: Duration:

Sweet-Ass Affirmations

I am....

What are the two **most valuable actions**
I will take today to progress toward my
goals, dreams, and optimal health?

1.

2.

What makes me ☺ and why?

Wildcard

Knowledge Bomb

If you were stranded on a deserted island
with just one diabetic, who would it be?

(Answer: Tom Hanks)

Sweet-Ass Reward

How will I reward myself after accomplishing
my two valuable actions today?

My **wins** for the day are:

Party Checklist

☐ Rx ☐ Test ☐ Water
☐ Nutrition ☐ Movement ☐ Reward

Breath of Life

Close your eyes and breathe deeply for as long as possible.

Current Mood: Duration:

What are the two **most valuable actions** I will take tomorrow to
progress toward my goals, dreams, and optimal health?

1.

2.

Sweet-Ass Affirmations

I am....

Reflection and Thoughts

You are **96** % done with optimizing your diabetic lifestyle. ☺   **BG:**

DATE .... / .... / 20 ....

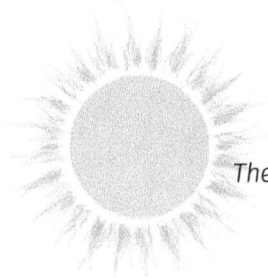

There will come a time when you think everything is finished.
That will be the beginning.
– Louis L' Amour

BG:

Breath of Life

Close your eyes and breathe deeply for as long as possible.

Current Mood: Duration:

Sweet-Ass Affirmations

I am....

What are the two **most valuable actions** I will take today to progress toward my goals, dreams, and optimal health?

1.

2.

What makes me ☺ and why?

Wildcard

Disconnect Challenge

Today, if you are tempted to watch television or browse the internet, try replacing it with reading a book or taking a walk outside instead.

Sweet-Ass Reward

How will I reward myself after accomplishing my two valuable actions today?

My **wins** for the day are:

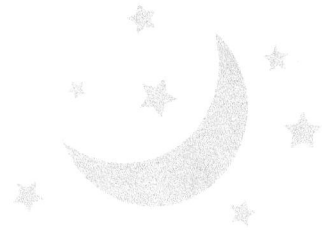

Party Checklist

☐ Rx   ☐ Test   ☐ Water

☐ Nutrition   ☐ Movement   ☐ Reward

Breath of Life

Close your eyes and breathe deeply for as long as possible.

Current Mood: Duration:

What are the two **most valuable actions** I will take tomorrow to progress toward my goals, dreams, and optimal health?

1.

2.

Sweet-Ass Affirmations

I am....

Reflection and Thoughts

You are   **97** % done with optimizing your diabetic lifestyle. ☺   **BG:**

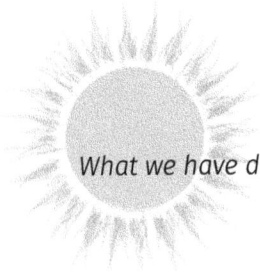

DATE .... / .... / 20 ....

What we have done for ourselves dies within us. What we have done for others and the world remains and is immortal.
– Albert Pike

BG:

Breath of Life

Close your eyes and breathe deeply for as long as possible.

Current Mood: Duration:

Sweet-Ass Affirmations

I am....

What are the two **most valuable actions** I will take today to progress toward my goals, dreams, and optimal health?

1.

2.

What makes me ☺ and why?

Wildcard

Abundance List

I have an abundance of:

Sweet-Ass Reward

How will I reward myself after accomplishing my two valuable actions today?

My **wins** for the day are:

Party Checklist

☐ Rx   ☐ Test   ☐ Water

☐ Nutrition   ☐ Movement   ☐ Reward

Breath of Life

Close your eyes and breathe deeply for as long as possible.

Current Mood: Duration:

What are the two **most valuable actions** I will take tomorrow to progress toward my goals, dreams, and optimal health?

1.

2.

Sweet-Ass Affirmations

I am....

Reflection and Thoughts

You are **98** % done with optimizing your diabetic lifestyle. ☺   **BG:**

DATE .... / .... / 20 ....

You're alive. If that's not something to smile about,
then I don't know what is.
– Chad Sugg

BG:

Breath of Life

Close your eyes and breathe deeply for as long as possible.

Current Mood: Duration:

Sweet-Ass Affirmations

I am....

What are the two **most valuable actions** I will take today to progress toward my goals, dreams, and optimal health?

1.

2.

What makes me ☺ and why?

Wildcard

Knowledge Bomb

Diabetes is not just about your medication or the food you consume. It is also about loving yourself, and finding things to praise, rather than criticize. You are doing AMAZINGLY well.

Sweet-Ass Reward

How will I reward myself after accomplishing my two valuable actions today?

My **wins** for the day are:

Party Checklist

☐ Rx   ☐ Test   ☐ Water

☐ Nutrition   ☐ Movement   ☐ Reward

Breath of Life

Close your eyes and breathe deeply for as long as possible.

Current Mood: Duration:

What are the two **most valuable actions** I will take tomorrow to
progress toward my goals, dreams, and optimal health?

1.

2.

Sweet-Ass Affirmations

I am....

Reflection and Thoughts

You are **99**% done with optimizing your diabetic lifestyle. ☺   **BG:**

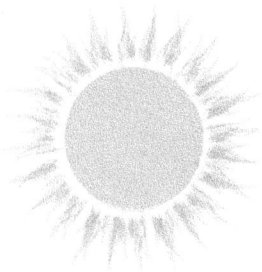

DATE .... / .... / 20 ....

Don't cry because it's over. Smile because it happened.
– Dr. Seuss

BG:

Breath of Life

Close your eyes and breathe deeply for as long as possible.

Current Mood: Duration:

Sweet-Ass Affirmations

I am....

What are the two **most valuable actions** I will take today to progress toward my goals, dreams, and optimal health?

1.

2.

What makes me ☺ and why?

Wildcard

Giving Challenge

What will I give today to impact someone's life in a positive way?

Sweet-Ass Reward

How will I reward myself after accomplishing my two valuable actions today?

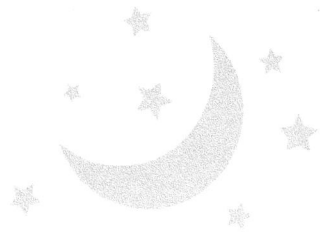

My **wins** for the day are:

Party Checklist

☐ Rx ☐ Test ☐ Water

☐ Nutrition ☐ Movement ☐ Reward

Breath of Life

Close your eyes and breathe deeply for as long as possible.

Current Mood: Duration:

What are the two **most valuable actions** I will take tomorrow to progress toward my goals, dreams, and optimal health?

1.

2.

Sweet-Ass Affirmations

I am....

Reflection and Thoughts

You are **100** % done with optimizing your diabetic lifestyle. ☺

BG:

Sweet-Ass Finish Line

YEEEEEEHAAAAAWWWW! YOU DID IT! You beautiful maniac! You defeated your resistance gremlins and finished your 100-day journey to optimize your diabetic lifestyle!

How does it feel? What has changed in your life? Did the visions you set at the beginning of the journey manifest? Take a moment to sit back and reflect on the last 100 days of journaling, and notice the difference between the person you are now, and the person you were when you started.

What were the highlights of your journey? What were the most memorable takeaways for you?

Go back through your journal and read your entries. That warm, fuzzy feeling will overwhelm you. Notice the people you have touched through the kindness of your gifts, and also the acceleration and growth of your wins!

It's important to celebrate and reward yourself for your accomplishment! Do something you've always wanted to do. Skydiving? Backpacking across another country? Pogo-sticking across the neighborhood in your undies? Anything! (We will not take responsibility if you get arrested for pogo-sticking in your undies.)

Needless to say, we are infinitely proud of you, not just because you completed your journal, but because you supported and fought for your wild, crazy, and "unrealistic" lifestyle and dreams.

We respect you and salute you. We worked so hard to create a fun system that would have everlasting impact on your approach to life, and we hope that you were able to create habits that will exponentially grow into infinite happiness, freedom, and purpose, forever.

Whether you realize it or not, the energy of your transformation has directly planted seeds in others around you to help awaken their own journeys.

Your next 100 days start whenever you are ready! Let's party like diabetics!

Sweet-Ass Vision Final Review

After 100 sweet-ass days of journaling, what kind of progress did you make towards bringing your visions to life? It's time to reflect on your journey and the ongoing relevance of your visions!

Below, take a moment to write out your three visions. Remember to write them in the present or past tense, as if you are achieving or have already achieved them! Chances are, you have made significant progress in bringing your visions to reality. Celebrate!

It's extremely important to maintain, update, and continue to pursue your visions as you move forward. Keep your momentum rolling! Take some time to reflect and celebrate all that is magical in your life, then get ready for your next 100 day quest!

My sweet-ass visions are:

- ....

- ....

- ....

Everyday is a bonus round. Slow down and enjoy something beautiful!

Special Invitation to Connect

We would love to hear from you about your experience with this journal and practice. It is our great honor to share this part of us with you, and we hope you will take a few moments to share your experience with us.

You can email us at **partylikeadiabetic@gmail.com** or join the Facebook community group and meet other amazing people by accessing the resource links at: **www.sweetassjournal.com/pladbonus**

If you found value in this journal and practice, consider gifting it to family members, friends, and co-workers. It's always magical to watch the domino effect! If you want multiple copies, please hit us up via email and we can give you a bulk discount.

And lastly, subscribe to our Patreon community to get access to premium health tools, group/mastermind video calls, exclusive bonus content, and ongoing community support! We look forward to meeting you! Easy. Breezy. Diabeezy!

Access our Patreon party here: **www.sweetassjournal.com/pladpatreon**

Coaching / Personal Journeys

You have done such an incredible job! If you would like to continue with your progress toward your goals and optimal health, Caitlin offers one-on-one health coaching as well as group coaching focusing in areas such as stress management, mindfulness, time management, work-life balance, and motivation.

By working with her, you will continue to define and achieve your optimal health goals with unconditional support and accountability.

To learn more, visit
www.partylikeadiabetic.co
or email Caitlin at
partylikeadiabetic@gmail.com

To happiness and health!

Acknowledgments

Heath Armstrong

First, I'd like to thank the magical Universe for seeding my mind with infinite ideas and opportunities, and for gifting me with the most loving and supportive family, friends, and team in all of the intergalactic galaxies.

To Steven Pressfield for limitless inspiration. To my pup Sachi for pure love. To Jared Angaza, Jacqueline du Plessis, Amber Vilahuaer, Honoree Corder, Hal Elrod, Kim Nicol, Dave Lent, and Paul Kemp for the patience of guiding me in the beginning when I was face-down, pants-down in the bushes.

To Lily Fouts, Ray Blakney, JC Spears, and Tiffany Hunter for putting up with my over-dramatic rollercoaster of entrepreneur highs and lows in our weekly calls.

To Jason Berwick and Alf-Jam Kelly, for being my best friends and understanding the risk and reward of the game.

And to Caitlin Grenier, for this beautiful collaboration and all of your vibrant energy. You are doing miraculous work, and I'm honored to have created this with you.

Caitlin Grenier

To my amazing parents. Words cannot describe how grateful I am for your unconditional love and support which encourages me every day to live my purpose. Without you this would not be possible.

To my sister Rachel without whom Party Like I ike A Diabetic would not exist! Thank you for serving as an inspiration and helping me realize that I can make a big difference in the world.

To Shandra, for your love, honesty, support, and unwavering friendship throughout everything. To Shelly, for always being there to talk through ideas and lovingly talking me off the edge (many times). To Jenna, for going through hell and back with me only to come out stronger on the other side.

To all of my diabuddies for inspiring me to stay strong, to keep fighting, and to live my best life.

Last, but certainly not least, to Heath. Thank you for helping my dream come true. You are truly changing the world.

OTHER PROJECTS

More from Heath Armstrong:

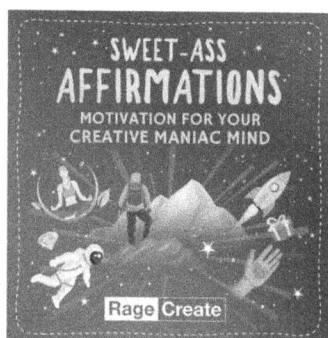

Sweet-Ass Affirmations
Motivation for Your Creative Maniac Mind.

60 witty, thought-provoking affirmation cards paired with bursts of motivation to help motivate your creative maniac mind!

Available on **RageCreate.com** and **Amazon.com**

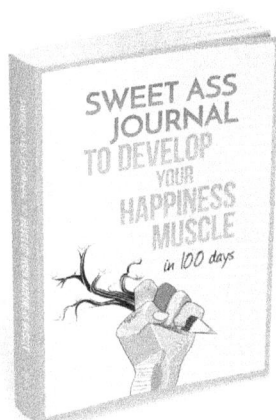

The Sweet Ass Journal to Develop Your Happiness Muscle in 100 Days (2017 Edition)

Destroy all resistance gremlins that attack you and manifest your visions in 100 days! The Sweet Ass Journal is a 100-day guided journal which walks you through the power of setting visions, practicing gratitude, idea generation, focus action, giving gifts, eliminating distractions, celebrating wins, planning, meditation, and reflection. It's a non-overwhelming, witty adventure that has been celebrated by freedom warriors all over the world!

The journal is available on **Amazon.com**

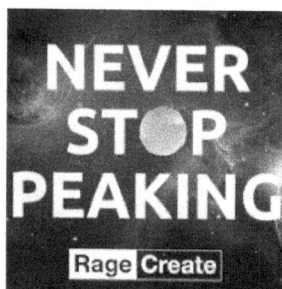

The Never Stop Peaking Podcast

The Never Stop Peaking Podcast is a cosmic exploration of higher development within the mind, heart, gut, and environment. I facilitate and channel conversations, stories, and media to dissect the purpose and magic of optimal health, habitual patterns, psychedelics, sacred plant medicines, authentic relatability, flow, nomadic journeys, energetic synchronicities, and the beautiful collective consciousness of our being.

Available on **iTunes** / **Stitcher** / **Google Play** / **Spotify** & More

More from Caitlin Grenier

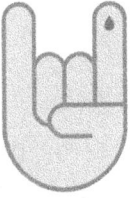

Party Like A Diabetic

An online platform that provides carb counts and menu substitutions for the most loved local food and drink venues in Tennessee, Hawaii, Alaska, Oregon, Arizona, and Colorado. If you would like your favorite spots to be listed, send me a message!

PartyLikeADiabetic.co

Follow the Party on Social Media:

Instagram: @partylikeadiabetic
Facebook: facebook.com/partylikeadiabetic
LinkedIn: linkedin.com/in/caitlin-grenier-127608114

About the Author - Heath Armstrong

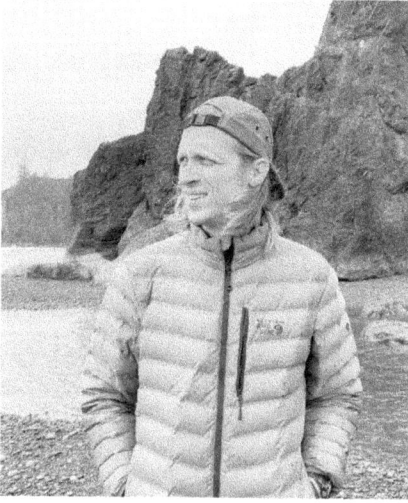

Heath Armstrong is a Serial Creative Maniac, Resistance Gremlin Smasher, and the Author of The Sweet-Ass Journal to Develop Your Happiness Muscle in 100 Days. In under 4 years, he interviewed 100+ creative entrepreneurs around the world on habits that made them successful, quit his job, sold all of his belongings, and created an e-commerce business that has generated more than $2 million in sales to date. He is also the host of The Never Stop Peaking Podcast, and the co-creator and author of Sweet-Ass Affirmations: Motivation for Your Creative Maniac Mind.

@heathfistpumps / **www.heatharmstrong.com**

About the Author - Caitlin Grenier

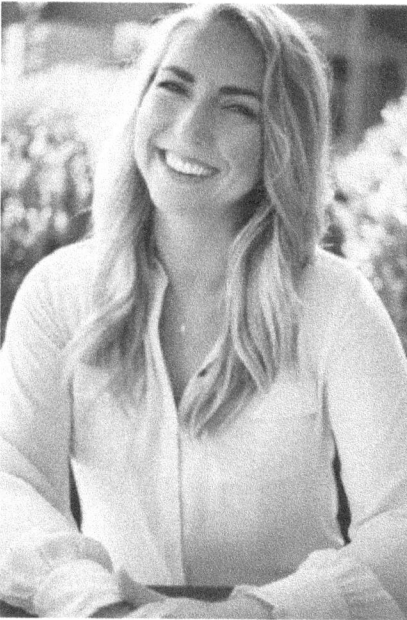

Caitlin Grenier is a National Board Certified Health and Wellness Coach and Founder of Party Like A Diabetic. After being diagnosed with late-onset type 1 diabetes in 2013, she decided to make the best out of her "new normal" and help others do the same. After growing up in Alaska and Hawaii, Caitlin is now living in Nashville, Tennessee. When she isn't traveling (which is rare) she enjoys dancing, concerts, volleyball, reading, sports, and her pet succulent "Sherman". In addition to coaching and growing PLAD, she is an adjunct instructor at Meharry Medical College where she teaches foundational health coaching skills and communication to medical students. She is also on the Community Leadership Board for the Middle Tennessee American Diabetes Association.

@partylikeadiabetic / **www.partylikeadiabetic.co**

www.ingramcontent.com/pod-product-compliance
Lightning Source LLC
Chambersburg PA
CBHW080556030426
42336CB00019B/3205